Medicine in Crisis
A Christian Response

edited by

Ian L. Brown and Nigel M. de S. Cameron

RUTHERFORD HOUSE BOOKS
Edinburgh

Published by Rutherford House,
17 Claremont Park, Edinburgh EH6 7PJ, Scotland

ISBN 0 946068 23 2 (casebound)
ISBN 0 946068 24 0 (limp)

Computer typeset at Rutherford House on Apple Macintosh Plus.
Printed by Chong Moh, Singapore.

CONTENTS

CONTRIBUTORS

The Revd Dr Nigel M. de S. Cameron is Warden of Rutherford House, Edinburgh.

The Revd James Philip is Minister of Holyrood Abbey Church, Edinburgh.

Dr Susan M. Holloway is a Research Fellow at the University of Edinburgh Human Genetics Unit.

The Revd David Easton is Minister of Burnside Parish Church, Glasgow.

Miss Pamela F. Sims is Consultant in Obstetrics and Gynaecology, Hexham.

Dr Ian L. Brown is Lecturer in Pathology and Consultant Pathologist, Western Infirmary, Glasgow.

Dr George L. Chalmers is Consultant in Administrative Charge, Glasgow East District Geriatrics Service.

PREFACE

Time was, as has been said, when medical ethics was discussed 'by consultants, with consultants and in private'. But times have changed, and for two fundamental reasons.

First, medicine has changed – of that there can be no doubt. The ethical ground-rules of a hundred generations have been set aside, and abortion and euthanasia are suddenly acceptable – in the eyes of many. This is hardly the fault of medicine, since the doctors' values have simply followed those of their societies. But its significance can hardly be over-stated.

Secondly, the demands which we are making on medicine have changed too. The new ethical tone of our society has enabled a new technology to flourish, and we have come to expect services of the doctor which we never did before.

So medical ethics has come out of the closet, and it has never been more important for there to be a Christian response to what is going on. In a modest fashion, and focusing on some particular questions, that is what this volume sets out to do. But we must be under no illusions. The definition and defence of the Christian medical tradition is one of the great tasks that lies before the church. We must pray that the God who inspired that tradition and the selfless service of so many of its adherents will himself maintain it, in an increasingly selfish and godless society.

Nigel M. de S. Cameron
Rutherford House,
Edinburgh
October 9th, 1987

NEW MEDICINE FOR OLD?[1]

Nigel M. de S. Cameron

There can be few who would dispute today that medicine in the western world is in a state of crisis, and few among Christian commentators who would not see this crisis in medical values as an aspect of the general moral flux into which the west has fallen. To some extent, it represents the outworking in a particular discipline of the problems inherent in the general collapse of the Christian *Weltanschauung*. After many false dawns – or false sunsets, as perhaps we should say – it is hard not to believe that we are finally witnessing the beginning of the end of the 'Christian Era'. The system of belief which the mind of the west has now so steadfastly put behind it was the custodian of the value-system which is presently in the process of final unravelling. There is no institution or discipline inherited from our Christian past which will ultimately escape the consequences of the severing of its roots in the mind and the values of an intellectual and spiritual order which are now seen as those of another world.

But the salami slicing which has ended the Christian dominance of the mind of the west has not resulted in immediate catastrophe. Belief has been consciously abandoned, but it is only little by little that the tide of Christian values has begun to ebb. The conviction has been strongly held that values can survive when the theological system and religious experience which gave rise to them and once gave them meaning have departed. Needless to say, this is a sentiment of considerable comfort for a society which is steadily shedding its religious convictions. Like most such misapprehensions, its seeming veracity actually reflects a partial truth. A remarkable degree of inconsistency is possible between belief and conduct, in a community as in an indi-

---

1. A version of this chapter was delivered as the 1987 Annual Public Lecture of the Bible Training Institute, Glasgow.

vidual. The tenacious survival into the Christian centuries of an institution like slavery illustrates the blindness of which good men are capable. We need to realise that inconsistency works both ways, and that it is equally possible for us to be good when we have ceased, on our own admission, to have reason to be.

Why this should be so we can only guess: in this case it plainly represents the grace of God, using human inconsistency to preserve us from the deserved ethical consequences of our abandonment of faith. But it also serves to obscure the long-term changes in values and conduct which must inevitably follow from changes in conviction. At least, it does for a time. First in smaller, then in larger, ways the new order begins to break the surface. By then it is too late to pull back. The investment in fundamental religious and theological change, made long since, is finally paying its dividend. And the world will never be the same again.

Indeed, the most startling and also the most solemn of all the signs of the new order is that its appearing does not shock. Time was when even the enthusiasts of unbelief denied *ex animo* the ethical implications which their critics laid at their door. But when the time has come and the ugliest truth begins to be plain for all to see, they do not think it ugly, since their moral perception has been shifted as the values of the new order fall into place. It is the corruption of that perception which is perhaps the gravest of all the corruptions of the new order in medicine. That which would have provoked not so much dissent as outrage in a former generation has become merely commonplace, and taken its place among the ethical furniture. There is incomprehension among good and conscientious members of the profession as to how it could possibly cause offence. This incomprehension is the surest sign that the new medicine has finally arrived.

And yet, it has been a long time coming. Inertia in matters of institutional life and professional practice has led the values of the past to retain a remarkable hold on medicine, notwithstanding the fact that its members have largely dispensed with the intellectual substructure of those values in

2

Christian belief. Indeed, it is a feature of institutional life that it is possessed of a momentum which maintains its character long after its logic has passed. But with the passage of time, in the lives of individuals and in the lives of communities, the logic of fundamental commitments in faith and values asserts itself, and consistency is restored.

There are special factors operating in the case of the profound changes affecting the values of medicine: it is not simply another creature of the decay of the Christian mind.

First, it is the profession which has most plainly and most thoroughly mirrored the Christian values of the society in which it has developed. So it is under a special threat when that value-system begins to decay. There is a sense in which all the professions have imbibed the Christian value-system, since the idea of a profession brings with it a package of values which is distinctly, although perhaps not exclusively, Christian in character. In this sense, medicine may be seen as the most characteristic of all the professions. The notions of trust, confidence, service, respect which comprise the 'professional' virtues are embodied in medicine in a way in which they are nowhere else – at least, nowhere else in the secular, as opposed to the specifically ecclesiastical, domain. The crisis in medicine as its values are severed from their Christian roots is the greater since, as it were, it has grown so tall.

Secondly, the chief value in our inherited practice of medicine is incommensurate with all other values. From its first beginnings among the Hippocratic physicians of ancient Greece, the humane medical tradition has set the sanctity of human life at the chief focus of its self-understanding. It is around this principle and from it that all other values have flowed. We may find it hard to imagine how, without it – with, let us say, a consistently utilitarian understanding of human life – the profession of medicine as we know it could ever have come to be. And it remains to be seen whether what we have come to cherish as an ethical discipline and not as a simple hiring of technical expertise, will survive departure from the Hippocratic principle.

Yet this particular principle, the keystone and coping-stone of medical values, is both the principal fruit of Christian anthropology and the principal casualty of its rejection. And it is in the repudiation of that anthropology that modern man's view of himself finds its chief characteristic. That is to say, the fundamental principle on which medicine has developed is at the heart of the Christian doctrine of man. The denial of that doctrine is the major tenet of the secular humanist, who in the blindness of his assertion that only man matters manages to deny that man matters at all, splendidly inverting the Christian conviction that man matters at all only because, finally, the only one who matters is God.

Thirdly, our society has assigned the doctor a role of constantly increasing importance. So at the very time that the logic of medicine as a coherent discipline is under threat, its scope and opportunity to impinge upon our experience and on the character of society as a whole are being enlarged. There are many reasons why this is so. At one level, as is widely recognised, the decline of the role of the clergy, and the break-up of the extended family, have left the doctor as an increasingly important figure in family and community. At the same time, changes in the values of society at large have placed new demands on the doctor: and it is here that the twin challenges of abortion and euthanasia – the taking of life before and after birth – find their place. Developments in medical technology, such as *in vitro* fertilisation, have posed new questions to which there are no longer old answers to give. Yet medicine faces these new challenges shorn of the values which would once have enabled it to cope with them.

The anatomy of the old medicine was an anatomy of healing. In the tradition of Hippocrates and the Judaeo-Christian values of western medicine, the doctor is a healer, no more and no less. The Hippocratic Oath bears this out in a number of interesting particulars, as medicine is defined by the drawing of its boundaries. The doctor is pledged to 'do no harm' to his patient as he seeks to do good. Lest this be misunderstood, the Oath goes on to repudiate those two acts in which the

4

doing of good and the doing of harm are confused. The Hippocratic physician forswears both abortion and euthanasia. For the 'first time in our tradition', as Margaret Mead has noted, there was 'a complete separation between curing and killing' in the rise of Hippocratic medicine.

The implication is unavoidable. If healing is difficult, indeed if it is altogether beyond the reach of the physician, he will not let go of his hold on the sanctity of his patient's life. There is no room left for short-circuiting the dilemma of treating the incurable. When medicine fails in its healing task, it cannot turn to another. These principles are the more striking when we place them in their context in ancient Greece, since in a primitive society – as, to a lesser degree, in more primitive medical situations today – the management options may be drastically limited, and the pressure to seek another way out when treatment fails to heal must be the stronger.

This pattern is being supplanted by one in which, in the place of 'healing', the chief end of the physician has become the 'relief of suffering'. At first sight the distinction may appear subtle. It is certainly true that in many cases the conduct of the physician will remain the same, whether he understands his role in classical, Hippocratic terms, or in those of the new medicine. That is so since in many cases the patient's suffering can best be relieved by his being healed. The fact of this practical coincidence of new medicine and old is one reason why many doctors are unable to see any distinction between the two.

How great a difference in principle lies behind such a convergence in practice begins to become evident when we note that the Hippocratic Oath itself does not even refer to the relief of suffering among the tasks of the physician. Since so much of his energy is directed to this end, the omission is curious. It is perhaps explicable in the light of the fundamental distortion which is brought about by the false elevation of this vital but subordinate task to the improper role in which it is found in the new medicine. For if it is not subordi-

5

nated to the healing role it inevitably challenges the principle of the sanctity of life.

And it is to underline this principle that the Oath insists that the physician renounce the taking of human life, the ultimate option in clinical management, and the only permanent solution, when restorative medicine has failed. The Hippocratic repudiation of abortion and euthanasia is the logical concomitant of the concept of the physician as healer. He is to heal and do no harm; he is *not* to relieve suffering at any price.

Yet the matter is not so simple as it seems. Having elevated the relief of suffering in the place of healing as the principal task of the physician, advocates of the new medicine argue that there is inevitable competition between this principle and the sanctity of life. The implication is that this competition is to be found in the life of an individual patient who is both suffering and incurable. But the programmatic significance of the 'relief of suffering' in the displacement of the old medicine by the new is properly evident only on a more candid examination of the way in which the values of the new medicine are beginning to operate. Two particular points must be made.

First, ever broader definitions of 'suffering' are employed. We may imagine a patient in incurable and unrelievable pain as the paradigm, but 'suffering' in this argument is in fact cross-referenced to the entire discussion about 'quality of life'. The 'relief of suffering' is code for 'the continuance of life of an unacceptable quality'. And whereas it is possible to mount a credible definition of 'suffering' understood in a narrow sense, in this broader context we find ourselves dealing in the undefinable (because necessarily subjective) concept of 'quality'. Yet, in this discussion, such a concept has to bear the weight of counter-balancing the principle of the sanctity of life. It is offered as a foil to sanctity conceived as an absolute, and the physician's handling of human life depends finally upon its adequacy.

Secondly, we must note that the paradigm of a patient's 'sufferings' raising problems for the sanctity of his or her own

6

life is misleading at another level also. It is common for abortion, for example, to be defended in just this way, yet here the 'suffering' is in most cases that of the *gravida* and the life at stake that of the *fetus*. It is in order to relieve her sufferings that the fetal life must be ended. The sanctity of one life is put in the balance with the suffering of another.

Less obviously, this weighing of the 'sufferings' of A against the life of B is evident also elsewhere. So in the case of the killing of deformed neo-nates, as in that of the dementing elderly, the *prima facie* argument is that the suffering/quality of life of the person concerned is such that relief is the duty of the physician. Yet it is rarely so simple. In almost every case there is a part played by the 'suffering' of the relatives, and the physician; and it is often the major part. Whatever may be said by physician and relatives alike – and, indeed, whatever may be honestly believed by them – there is often little actual interest in the calculus of pain and pleasure in the patient. Dementia involves a retreat into a private world in which the patient is content, however distressing others may find it. Down's Syndrome, as is well known, produces a typically happy and contented character. Yet those who suffer from these conditions are in the front line for euthanasia, both in ethical argument, and in informal but growing practice.

What is more, the concept of the 'suffering' of unknown future individuals or of society at large is increasingly considered relevant. It is already a dominant factor in the debate about the experimental use of human embryos, whose lives are held to be forfeit to the prevention of such 'suffering'. We explore this question in a later chapter, but it is relevant here to point out that the seeming dialectic of suffering and sanctity in a single life has here become the gateway to the use of human lives as means to ends.

We turn now to a related element in the justification of the new medicine, that of compassion. The new medicine claims as its fundamental principle a compassion which is superior to that of the tradition. Compassion is invoked as the supreme medical virtue, motivating and governing hu-

7

mane medical practice and displacing the cold principles of the tradition. In particular, it is contrasted with the sanctity of life, which is painted as an abstract concept which is the enemy and not the friend of the patient. The physician must let compassion be the over-riding determinant of his treatment.

This is a compelling argument, with its implication that by elevating the principle of the sanctity of life the tradition of Hippocrates has lacked compassion and therefore been less than complete in virtue. Indeed, the picture is drawn of a heartless tradition, and its implication is that those who maintain it or defend it today are ethically deficient. The moral case is that of the new, more humane medicine in which compassion is untrammelled by such abstractions as sanctity. The problem is that such a claim rests upon a confusion. For compassion on its own is neither virtue nor vice; it is an emotion. The invocation of compassion *in this argument* is – wittingly or not – a cover for the ethic which lies behind it, the ethic which denies the sanctity of life. Compassion is a fellow-feeling with someone who is suffering. Its effect is to catalyse action to meet their need, and in that sense could be said to be virtuous. But it catalyses action in line with ethical principles which have already been decided, and which may accordingly be of any kind, good or bad. And in some cases it can lead to action which is morally reprehensible. Such is the compassion (which may be real enough) of the abortionist. The new medicine has no monopoly of compassion. It has been the motive power of the Hippocratic tradition. The difference lies not between a compassionate medicine and an uncompassionate, but between a compassion which will not let go of the sanctity of human life, and a compassion which will – in the interests of some perceived greater good.

Indeed, we may go further and suggest that if compassion, as the supreme motivation for medicine, breaks free from the sanctity of life, its ground will ultimately be eroded, for the dignity of the patient is finally inseparable from the sanctity of his or her life. The suggestion, therefore, that the

8

new medicine is more compassionate than the old is without foundation. It is, in effect, the substitution of one compassion for another; but compassion free of sanctity is the proper motivation not of human but of veterinary medicine.

The difficulty with attempted qualifications of the sanctity of human life is that it is an absolute principle, and therefore strictly incapable of qualification. If qualified, it is lost, and some other – lesser – principle must stand in its place. The contrast with another phrase which has lately gained wide currency, 'respect for life', is striking . Of course, human life is to be respected, and there are entirely proper uses of this phrase. It is because human life is possessed of sanctity that it is to be respected, and seen thus as an implication of sanctity it states an important principle. But it can also be used otherwise, as a substitute for sanctity, and it is increasingly used in this way. Respect can be qualified as sanctity cannot, and can be set in some other place in the hierarchy of values than at the apex. With sanctity this is not so. If it has any place at all – if it is a statement of something that is true – then it can have no place other than at the apex of our ethics. And below it there is room for the other principles of the old medicine, room for healing, for suffering to be relieved, for medicine to be practised within the boundaries of Hippocrates: no abortion, no euthanasia – no taking of human life – no harm. Without it, it is hard to see what ground there lies for any concept of respect which gives effect to the recognition of human life as uniquely valuable; hard to see what final motive remains for a medicine that is dedicated first and last to the interests of the patient.

Which is to say that the old medicine is a package, tied together with its doctrine of life's sacred and inviolable quality. The new medicine is another, whose final shape and character remain to be discovered. Yet we would be mistaken to believe that the new medicine will finally prove to be no more than a re-issue of the old – more open, compassionate and realistic but recognisably the same. Whatever its advocates and practitioners claim, and may indeed believe, the shift from 'sanctity' to 'respect' has been momentous. Its implications have barely begun to be visible, and though we shall shortly turn to a survey of the 'life issues' in which the clash of old and new has so far been so evident, we would be less than candid if we confined our discussion to these questions (which form the major concerns of the essays to follow).

For, in truth, these questions are but illustrations of the fundamentally changed relationship of the physician to his patient. In the old medical tradition it was pre-eminently a relationship of service. In the new, it is one of power. And, while there have been other pressures at work beside the shift from 'sanctity' to 'respect' (the consequences, like this shift itself, of the general abandonment of the theological warrants for the sanctity of life, *viz*, the Christian view of God and man), it is in this shift itself that we see the essential explanation of this changed relationship. In the old medicine the patient was possessed of an absolute dignity, expressed in the sacrosanct quality of his or her life. However poor or degenerate or diseased the patient might be, the physician was committed to the ideal of disinterested service, since in his care was one who bore the divine image. Which is not to say that every physician within the tradition, or even most physicians, have lived up to their ideal: simply that this *was* their ideal, and *as an ideal* it is now being supplanted by another.

Once the shift from 'sanctity' to 'respect' has taken place, the entire picture has changed. For 'respect', when made to do duty for 'sanctity', is an inherently subjective concept. It is ironical that this term, which seems to honour the dignity of the respected subject, in fact dishonours him by denying the absolute character of his right to exist. His continued human life becomes a matter of medical decision-making, with a decision to end that life a management option for the physician. In practical terms, while the morality of sanctity brought with it a fundamental policy of 'do no harm', in the new medicine of respect this is no longer so. It is open to the physician to conclude that he will best 'respect' his patient by ending his life. Indeed, as in our discussion of the relief of

10

suffering, it is immediately evident that the morality of respect permits the physician to turn his attention from his patient to others, and to take account of their interests, as he perceives them, which may conflict with the interests of the patient; or, rather, which may coalesce with his perception of the patient's real interests and lead him to opt for the ending of his patient's life, out of 'respect' to all concerned. 'Respect for life' as an alternative to sanctity not only enables the physician to make such a judgement, but forces on him the necessity of these very choices on each occasion, whichever way he may decide. In the context of competing value-systems in which the medical profession finds itself today, the tendency will be (as we have suggested above) for those who embrace the principles of the new medicine still to arrive at the conclusions of the old. But this should not mislead us – or them – into believing that this is how the new medicine will always operate. When the physician takes the conservative option in such a situation he is being untrue to the new medicine, but he is still illustrating the change which has come upon medicine by having to make the choice. What is crucially new is that, irrespective of the outcome, such a decision was never faced in this way in the old medical tradition.

The grounding of the old medicine in the absolute character of the life of the patient secured for medical practice a tradition of service, the expertise of the physician always at the disposal of the patient and never set over against him and his interests. In its place, the new medicine is giving birth to a tradition of power, with the patient's actual interests open to subjective construction and, in effect, the patient at the physician's disposal rather than *vice versa*. This has many implications, particularly in increasingly pluralist societies where concepts of 'interests' and 'respect' are increasingly controverted, and where there is a growing tendency for the state to impose its own – even more secular – values upon its citizens. But its plainest implications have already become evident in the basic issues of life and death in which medicine is involved, the questions of abortion and euthanasia which are discussed at some length below. 'Curing' and 'killing', in the new medicine, are once more under the same head, options for the same physician, alternative responses to the patient. And those at the margins of society – the unborn, the handicapped new-born, and the elderly – are the first among the victims of this reversion to a medical tradition which, although new, is also very old. The pagan ethical principles of Hippocrates, so happily married with the Judaeo-Christian doctrine of man have, it seems, run their course. It may be many years before their influence on medicine finally fades, such is the human capacity to be eclectic and inconsistent. But it is now needful for the Christian to realise that the ethics of the profession are no longer the ethics of the church, and begin to consider the implications of Christian medicine in a post-Christian society which is unsurprisingly marked by post-Christian and post-Hippocratic medicine. As the crisis deepens and the character of our medical tradition continues to change, there can be no greater need than to maintain and develop a Christian medicine that is distinguished by its adherence to its own values. This role is unlikely to be popular, since the continued existence of Christian medicine will be seen as a threat to the new medical values of the majority, giving the lie to their claim of continuity with the Hippocratic tradition. It will also involve the development of a new consciousness on the part of Christian physicians who have grown accustomed to the general confluence of Christian and professional values, and who will increasingly discover fundamental divergences, and indeed conflict, between the two.

Indeed, some have already found it impossible to come to terms with the prophetic and dissident role which Christian medicine is being called to play, preferring to accept piecemeal elements of the new medicine in the hope that they can be harmonised with the old. But as time passes the divergence of new and old will become yet clearer; as in some areas, such as that of abortion, it has already become quite plain. To that extent the crisis in medicine is also a crisis in Christian medicine, as basic ethical choices are forced on members of the profession, and as the communal values of medical organisations increasingly shift out of line with the tradition and into line with the new ethics.

The old axis of sanctity-of-life and healing is rapidly being replaced by a new one of quality-of-life and relief-of-suffering. The change is one of historic importance, and the challenge to Christians in the medical and allied professions is the greatest they have faced in modern times. If they are to meet it, they must begin by recognising that medical ethical debates today are not chiefly about particular matters, important though they may be, but about the character of medicine as a whole. Is it to remain the discipline that we have known, the old medicine of Hippocrates and the Christian tradition, or will it become the new?

THE SANCTITY OF LIFE:
THE CHRISTIAN CONSENSUS

James Philip

The concern of this chapter is to underline and define the teaching of Scripture on the sanctity of life, and to show how deeply imbedded this idea is in the very presuppositions underlying the whole biblical revelation. It will be sufficient for our purpose to confine our line of enquiry to a threefold consideration: first of all, the theological implications of the doctrine of creation and particularly of man's creation in the image of God; then, the underlying assumptions of the Mosaic legislation, particularly in the book of Deuteronomy; and thirdly, the taking over of these in the New Testament, in the teaching of Jesus and of the Apostles, in the emphasis on the commandment to love, the teaching on 'the powers that be', and the recognition that life is a stewardship committed to all men, to be given account of, a stewardship reinforced by the doctrine of redemption: 'You are not your own, for you are bought with a price: therefore glorify God in your body and in your spirit, which are God's' (1 Cor. 6:19,20).

I

'And God said, Let us make man in our image, in our likeness . . . . So God created man in his own image, in the image of God created he him; male and female created he them' (Gen. 1:26,27). Such is the biblical testimony. The implications and importance of this seminal statement for the idea of the sanctity of life can hardly be over-estimated. It is essentially in virtue of the fact of being the creation of God that man's life is sacred: nothing made by God, and particularly nothing made in his image can be violated or desecrated with impunity.

It is not possible to read the sublime account of man's creation in Genesis without recognising that it had a distinctive place in the mind of God. It was not only the climax of his creative work, but it also shows the wonder of his goodness and love. It was after the creation of the world in all its glory and beauty that man was brought into being by divine deliberation. It is impressive and moving to see how God prepared everything in creation before he brought man, the crown of that creation, into existence.

What it means to say that man was made 'in the image of God' has been interpreted variously down the ages of Church history. The Reformers agreed with the early Fathers in holding that the image of God in man consisted primarily in man's rational and moral characteristics, and maintained that 'original righteousness' belonged to the very nature of man. In Calvin's words,

> By this term ('image of God') is denoted the integrity with which Adam was endued when his intellect was clear, his affections subordinated to reason, all his senses duly regulated, and when he truly ascribed all his excellence to the admirable gifts of his Maker. And though the primary seat of the divine image was in the mind and the heart, or in the soul and its powers, there was no part even of the body in which some rays of glory did not shine.[1]

This basic position which has been held to include not only the elements of true knowledge, righteousness and holiness but also those which belonged to the natural constitution of man – intellectual power, natural affections and moral freedom – has been elaborated in different ways. One scholar says: 'The image of God consists in that man, as a spiritual and moral being, gives expression, in a creaturely manner, to the inward characteristics of God'.[2] Another speaks of the image in terms of a reflection in a mirror, suggesting a correspondence rather than a resemblance between man and God. What is suggested in this interpretation is that man is created for communion with God, and that this is not merely an

1. Calvin, *Commentary* on Genesis 1:26.
2. G. F. Hendry, *The Westminster Confession of Faith*.

option that he may exercise or not as he so wills, but belongs to the basic structure of his existence.

All this has significance in relation to the biblical doctrine of the Fall of man, by which the image of God in man was defaced. It is important to have a proper understanding of the nature of this 'defacement' of the divine image. A useful and helpful way of coming to such an understanding is to recognise that the image of God in man must be considered in two ways, the *formal* and the *material*. As Brunner puts it:

> The formal sense of the concept is the human, i.e. that which distinguishes man from all the rest of creation, whether he be a sinner or not. Even the Old Testament speaks of man's likeness to God in this sense. It signifies above all the superiority of man within creation. Man has not, even as a sinner, ceased to be the central and culminating point of creation. This superior position in the whole of creation, which man still has, is based on his special relation to God, *i.e.* on the fact that God has created him for a special purpose - to bear his image. This *function* or calling as a bearer of the image is not only not abolished by sin; rather is it the presupposition of the ability to sin and continues within the state of sin.[3]

This *formal* aspect of the image of God above all emphasises that it belongs to the very nature of man to be a *responsible* being. This is a constant in his experience. Even as a sinner man remains responsible. This aspect of the image of God is something he does not, and cannot lose, but is entirely unaffected by sin. Man does not become an animal, or inanimate, through his sin, but remains a human being, responsible to God.

The *material* aspect of the image of God, however - that which consists in man's 'original righteousness' - is completely lost through sin; man is a sinner through and through, and there is nothing in him which is not defiled by sin. Furthermore, man loses, by his sin, 'all ability of will to any spiritual good accompanying salvation',[4] to use the words of

3. E. Brunner and Karl Barth, *Natural Theology*, London, 1946, p. 23.
4. *Westminster Confession of Faith*, 9:3.

the *Westminster Confession of Faith.* This means that, being dead in sins, he is unable to do anything to help himself or prepare himself for salvation. That is to say, through sin man has lost his freedom, and is no longer free to realise his divine destiny. But loss of freedom is not the same as loss of responsibility. Man as sinner is no longer a free agent, he is no longer able *not* to sin; but he does not thereby cease to be a responsible being; he remains unalterably responsible for his sin although he is no longer free to stop committing it. This is the tragic paradox that makes redemption so urgently necessary.

Such are the basic presuppositions underlying the biblical emphasis upon the sanctity of life and the inherent dignity of mankind, even in its wretchedness and sin, for it is made clear that man has not, even as a sinner, ceased to be the central and culminating point of creation. The reality of this idea is writ large on the pages of Scripture, and from its earliest beginnings. In the story of Cain and Abel in the opening chapters of Genesis we have indications of the sanctity attaching to man's life, and of the wrong involved in the taking of one man's life by another (Gen. 4). God's judgement on the violation of that sanctity is plainly indicated. Furthermore, the indication in that remarkable story is that life is so sacred that even the life of the murderer is to be respected, and not wantonly taken away (Gen. 4:15). This is not, as might first appear, an argument against the punishment of the guilty, nor an argument against capital punishment; rather, it is a prohibition against wanton revenge. As Keil and Delitzsch put it, 'From the very first God determined to take punishment into His own hands, and protect human life from the passion and wilfulness of human vengeance'.[5] That there can be no thought of waiving the punishment of the wicked here is made abundantly clear in the impressive statement in Genesis 9:5,6 about the protection of life made to Noah and his sons after the Flood: 'For your lifeblood I

5. Keil and Delitzsch on Genesis 4:15, *Commentary on the Old Testament*, vol. 1, p. 115.

will surely require a reckoning; of every beast I will require it and of man; of every man's brother I will require the life of man. Whoever sheds the blood of a man, by man shall his blood be shed; for God made man in his own image.'

Very significantly, the idea of the sanctity and sacredness of life clearly implicit in these words is based on the fact that man is made in the image of God. It is also important to realise that in these words, in contrast to those in Genesis 4, where God indicated that punishment would be kept in his own hands, he now delegates his authority in inflicting the punishment to man himself: 'By man shall his blood be shed' - thus placing in the hand of man his own judicial power. As Luther says, 'This was the first command having reference to the temporal sword. By these words temporal government was established, and the sword placed in its hand by God'.[6] Keil and Delitzsch comment thus:

> Hence the command does not sanction revenge, but lays the foundation for the judicial rights of the divinely appointed 'powers that be' (Rom. 13:1). This is evident from the reason appended: 'for in the image of God made he man'. If murder was to be punished with death because it destroyed the image of God in man, it is evident that the infliction of the punishment was not to be left to the caprice of individuals, but belonged to those alone who represent the authority and majesty of God, *i.e.* the divinely appointed rulers ... this command then laid the foundation for all civil government ... and the foundation for a well ordered civil development of humanity ....[7]

II

A great deal of misunderstanding exists as to the nature of Old Testament Scripture and how it is to be understood and interpreted. It is frequently assumed that much of the Mosaic legislation is not only legalistic in character, but harsh, pitiless and barbaric, particularly in contrast to the New

6. Luther, quoted by Keil and Delitzsch on Genesis 9:5,6, *ibid.,* p. 153.
7. Keil and Delitzsch, *ibid.,* p. 153.

Testament emphasis on love in the teaching of Jesus. One can only assume that such criticisms are either based on ignorance of the text of the Old Testament itself - who could fail to sense the heartbeat of divine love and compassion in such passages as, for example, Psalm 103:8-18, Isaiah 49:14-16, Jeremiah 31:1ff, Hosea 11:1ff, 14:1ff? - or that they are the fruit of an outdated liberal interpretation of Scripture alien to true biblical exegesis and long since abandoned by reputable scholarship. It will not do to cite our Lord's words in the Sermon on the Mount (Matt. 5-7) as evidence that he contradicted the allegedly harsh teaching of the Old Testament in favour of a 'truly Christian' position, for the simple reason that he was intent upon correcting, not the law itself ('I am not come to destroy but to fulfil') but the false, legalistic misinterpretation of the law placed upon it by the Pharisees of his day. It was their understanding of the law that was at fault; it was they, not he, who were at odds with the law. And a similar misunderstanding persists today in the contemporary attitude to the Mosaic legislation.

In point of fact, much of that legislation, in Leviticus, and particularly in Deuteronomy, manifests a remarkable spirit of tenderness and compassion, and above all - and this is central to our main consideration - a concern for the dignity and sanctity of human life. To take but one example: in Deuteronomy 21, we find an interesting selection of ordinances and regulations - the expiation of an uncertain murder (1-9), the treatment of a captive wife (10-14), the rights of the firstborn (15-17), the punishment of a refractory son (18-21), the burial of a hanged criminal (22,23). It may well be asked what the significance of these seemingly random laws might be. Keil and Delitzsch make the comment:

> The reason for grouping together these five laws, which are apparently so different from one another, as well as for attaching them to the previous regulations, is to be found in the desire to bring out

distinctly the sacredness of life and of personal rights from every point of view, and impress it upon the covenant nation.[8]

In another place the same commentators, in summing up a larger section of Deuteronomy, of which this chapter forms a part (chapters 19-26) give the following analysis:

> (Moses) seeks to establish upon a permanent basis the civil and domestic well-being of the whole congregation and its individual members, by a multiplicity of precepts, intended to set before the people, as a conscientious obligation on their part, reverence and holy awe in relation to human life, to property, and to personal rights; a pious regard for the fundamental laws of the world; sanctificaton of domestic life and of the social bond; practical brotherly love towards the poor, the oppressed, and the needy; and righteousness of walk and conversation.[9]

Some brief details of exposition of the enactments contained in this chapter will serve to substantiate this interpretation. As to the anonymous murder (1-9), such a murder, as the Tyndale Commentary points out 'involved the whole community in blood guilt. Both the people and the land were defiled, and some kind of ceremonial execution was required to satisfy the demands of justice'.[10] There is considerable significance in this. It is the sanctity of life that required and validated this symbolic 'death penalty' - the sacrifice of the animal - and demanded the infliction of it. As John Murray well says, 'The deeper our regard for life the firmer will be our hold upon the penal sanction which the violation of that sanctity merits'.[11] And Derek Kidner makes a similar point, in describing the imposition of the death penalty for murder:

8. Keil and Delitzsch on Deut. 21, *Commentary on the Old Testament*, vol. 3, p. 404.
9. Keil and Delitzsch, on Deut. 12-26, *op. cit.*, p. 351.
10. J. A. Thompson, *Commentary on Deuteronomy*, London, 1974, p. 225.
11. John Murray, *Principles of Conduct*, London, 1957, p. 225.

'Such a judicial taking of a murderer's life is an *affirmation*, not a *denial*, of the sanctity of human life'.

In the case of the captive wife (10-14) the enactment breathes a spirit of humane and compassionate consideration, standing in marked contrast, as the Tyndale Commentary points out, 'with the cruel treatment meted out to women captives of war among the neighbouring nations'.[12] Once again, it is the basic idea of the sanctity of life which informs such a compassion.

A similar emphasis underlies the enactment of the rights of the firstborn (15-17). The reason why these could not be waived or set aside on mere human considerations, such as a father's personal preference for a favourite son, is that the firstborn, as the first-fruits of a marriage, belonged to God, and therefore any violation of the law concerning the firstborn would be regarded as an attack upon God and upon the sanctity of the life that had been set apart for him.

Even the case of the punishment of a refractory son (18-21), hard and severe as it may seem, bears the same message. What is stressed here is the importance of a stable family life: disobedience and rebelliousness threaten the sacredness of the divine order, and strike at society itself. The need to hold all the arrangements of God sacred, whether in nature or in social life, is ever the paramount consideration.

In the same way, the burial of an executed criminal (22,23), and the prohibition against leaving him hanging in the public gaze, were in all probability designed to draw the veil over the disgrace and shame done to a creature made in the image of God. The punishment was necessary, in order to affirm the sanctity of the life that had been taken by the murderer, but there was no doubt as to the fact that prolonged public exposure was regarded as violating the image. Calvin's comment on these verses is as follows:

> The object of this precept was to banish inhumanity and barbarism from the chosen people, and also to impress upon them horror even

12. J. A. Thompson, *op. cit.*, p. 228.

of a just execution . . . . Moses does not here speak generally, but
only of those malefactors who are unworthy of the honour of
burial; yet the public good is regarded in the burial even of such as
these, lest men should grow accustomed to cruelty, and thus become more ready to commit murder.[13]

Always, the emphasis is upon the sacredness, sanctity and
dignity of life, based - as we have seen in Genesis 9:6 - on
the fact that man is made in the image of God. This is the
uniform emphasis in the Old Testament, as innumerable
passages similar to those already quoted make plain.

III

One has only to make mention of the above considerations to
realise how substantially - and how dangerously - modern
attitudes have become detached from the biblical revelation
and the essential reverence for absolute values embedded in
it. Perhaps one of the most subtle and perilous assumptions
of all is to suppose that Jesus in his teaching disavowed Old
Testament notions on moral absolutes and advocated instead a spirit of compassion and love, and that 'human compassion' and the so-called 'humane' attitudes of modern
thinking are now the only worthy criteria, with anything differing from this to be regarded - and dismissed - as 'a
hangover from earlier times'.

We should not be blind to the terrible consequences in
modern society of such an attitude. One has only to mention
the steady and growing erosion of the principle of law and
order, and the emergence of a spirit of near anarchy, in social
and industrial life alike, which seems to be committed to the
acceleration of moral and spiritual decline in the nation; one
has only to think of the emergence into positions of strength
and influence of pressure groups of various kinds - minorities
of determined and dedicated men who exploit our democratic

13. Calvin, on Deut. 21:22, 23, *Harmony of the Four Last Books of the
Pentateuch*, p. 47.

freedoms for base and sinister ends, and who skilfully and ruthlessly manipulate public opinion through the mass media to such an extent that society has been 'conned' into regarding as normal and acceptable attitudes and patterns which even a few years ago would scarcely have been tolerated - to realise that the philosophy of so-called humanitarianism is, from the biblical point of view, the most inhuman and deadly of all 'isms' and ultimately destructive of the sanctity of human life as created in the image of God.

The success of such pressure groups, and the measure in which this evil philosophy has become all-pervasive, may be seen in the extent to which what someone has called 'the ethic of disposability' has permeated modern society: the divorce laws are relaxed, and 'humane' (!) legislation introduced in order to provide 'disposable marriage'; the 'abortion on demand' lobby, shrilly supported by the various 'rights' movements, is determined to establish the principle of 'disposable babies'; disclosures in the past few years about the practice of euthanasia or 'mercy-killing' have introduced the concept of 'disposable chronically sick and elderly people'.

The deadly implications of such thinking seem to be hidden from those who indulge it, or if not hidden, wilfully and culpably ignored; if it is legal and allowable to terminate human life, either in the womb, or in terminal illness, or in a geriatric ward, or simply in the case of someone who is tired of living and wants to die, it is not a very big step to make legal the termination of the life of someone *we* may want to die. Then, a time could come when a consensus of opinion - of 'humane, responsible' people, to be sure - would obtain in which it would be deemed that people over a certain age, or mentally disabled, or unable to live a 'meaningful' life, should be gently and quietly (and, of course, on humanitarian grounds) put down. We should beware of branding this as a fantastic and scare-mongering line of reasoning: for where moral absolutes are removed, such a development and progression is not only possible, but has in fact already been evident in modern times. The sombre history of Hitler's Nazi

Germany, which sent six million Jews into the gas chambers through such a philosophy, is a grim reminder of how far and to what extremes - and how quickly - such a road can lead.

The basic assumption that underlies all such dangerous thinking is that life is ours, to do with it what *we* choose. But it is this unwarrantable thesis that the biblical revelation so firmly disputes and denies. Life is *not* ours, in this sense, and never has been ours. It is given us as a stewardship from God. It belongs, in the last analysis, to him, and he alone has the disposal of it. This is also part of the meaning of the doctrine of man as made in the image of God, giving life a sanctity, and forbidding us to violate either others' lives or our own.

Not only is this emphasised in the teaching of the New Testament, in such explicit statements as the Pauline 'You are not your own, for you are bought with a price' (1 Cor. 6:19,20), a statement, it is true, having reference to our belonging to God by virtue of our redemption by Christ at the cost of his blood; it is also underlined unmistakeably in relation to mankind as a whole in such Old Testament passages as Daniel 5:23, in the words 'the God in whose hand your breath is, and *whose are all your ways*', words which are echoed implicitly in some of Christ's characteristic parables which deal with the idea of the stewardship of life and the giving account of that stewardship (cf. Matt. 18: 21-35, 25: 14-30, Lk. 16: 1-13).

It is the abandonment of this basic truth in modern thinking, and the substitution of so-called 'humanitarian' ideas - the discounting, so to speak, of the vertical relationship in favour of the horizontal - and therefore the severing of society's link with God - that has led to the emergence of such 'progressive' ideas. It is only in a society whose roots are no longer deep down in the principles of the biblical revelation that such thinking can ever flourish.

But we cannot afford to be taken in by fair-sounding and plausible talk about enlightened, liberal and humanitarian attitudes, for these have already opened a door that will be very difficult to close, and there is no saying what we will

24

see in our society within the next generation or two. What
we need are clear and unambiguous biblical attitudes based
on moral absolutes, and we must not fear that we shall be
either illiberal or unenlightened if we hold them. Modern
history, and all the available evidence from totalitarian
regimes, should serve to teach us that 'humane' and
'enlightened' theories have produced a fearful harvest of cruelty and inhumanity in the world, when they have been divorced from law and from God.

Dr Monk Gibbon's words, quoted by Arnold Lunn and
Garth Lean on the flyleaf of their book *The New Morality*,
provide an impressive and highly relevant conclusion to this
chapter:

> The truth is that civilization collapses when the essential reverence
> for absolute values which religion gives disappears. Rome had dis-
> covered that in the days of her decadence. Men live on the accumu-
> lated faith of the past as well as on its accumulated self-discipline.
> Overthrow these and nothing seems missing at first, a few sexual
> taboos, a little of the prejudice of a Cato, a few rhapsodical im-
> pulses - comprehensible, we are told, only in the literature of folk
> lore - these have gone by the board. But something has gone as
> well, the mortar which held society together, the integrity of the
> individual soul; then the rats come out of their holes and begin bur-
> rowing under the foundations and there is nothing to withstand
> them.[14]

14. Dr Monk Gibbon in *Mount Ida*, quoted by Lunn and Lean in *The
    New Morality*.

SCIENTIFIC DEVELOPMENTS: GENETIC ENGINEERING AND *IN VITRO* FERTILISATION

Susan M. Holloway

In this chapter two recent developments in biology and medicine will be discussed - namely, genetic engineering and *in vitro* fertilisation. A description of the present uses and possible future developments of each of these techniques will be given together with a discussion of some of the ethical issues raised. In conclusion, the Christian response to the introduction of these techniques will be considered.

Genetic Engineering

Genetic engineering has been described as the most revolutionary development in biology in recent years.[1] It can be described as the direct manipulation of the genetic material to determine its structure and function. Following on from this is the possibility of altering the genetic material in an intact organism and thus the characteristics of that organism.

In the past, attempts were made to improve the characteristics of living organisms by selective breeding. In *The Republic* Plato urged that in animal reproduction the best of both sexes should be brought together as often as possible and the worst allowed to come together as seldom as possible. The idea was to improve the quality of the flock. In the late nineteenth century Sir Francis Galton, a cousin of Charles Darwin, coined the word 'eugenics' for the hereditary improvement of man and animals by selective breeding.

In the present century the idea of the production of a super-race by selective breeding was taken up by Adolf Hitler. The hope was that the super-race would have characteristics which would predispose them to the role of leadership. Men and women were chosen as procreators of this race and

1. A. E. H. Emery, 'Recombinant DNA Technology', *Lancet*, 1981; ii:1406-9.

camps were set up in various countries outside Germany. However the experiment was a failure. The offspring had just as many ailments and shortcomings as children reared in the usual way.

With increasing knowledge of the mechanism of inheritance the fallacy of such experiments has been seen. However a new form of eugenics has begun to emerge. The idea is that the human race can be improved not by selective breeding but by genetic manipulation.

Present knowledge of the genetic material
Before proceeding to discuss genetic engineering in detail it is necessary briefly to summarize our current knowledge of the nature of the genetic material.

Within every cell of an animal or plant there is a nucleus containing a number of chromosomes. The exact number depends on the species concerned, but in man there are forty-six chromosomes in each cell. Arranged along the chromosomes are the genes which determine the structure of the proteins made in the cell. Each cell of the body contains an identical set of chromosomes but not every gene is functional in every cell and thus there are many different cell types.

In 1953 James Watson and Francis Crick made a discovery which was to revolutionize the science of genetics. They determined the chemical structure of the fundamental material of the chromosomes - deoxyribosenucleic acid (DNA). They demonstrated that DNA is in the shape of a long twisting double helix, each helix being composed of four types of sub-unit. DNA is reproduced by the separation of the two helices followed by the attraction of chemical substances to each single helix to produce two double helices as before.

In 1961 Dr Marshall Nirenberg showed that the ordering of the four sub-units of the DNA determined the structure of the proteins produced by the cell. Since that time it has been possible to map several hundred genes to specific chromosomes. Some genes have actually been synthesized from the four basic sub-units.

Susan M. Holloway

Recent developments in genetics
The most important recent development in genetics has been the introduction of recombinant DNA technology. The basic procedure is that fragments of DNA containing specific genes of interest are produced. Each is then incorporated into a suitable vector which is in turn introduced into a host organism, usually the bacterium *Escherichia coli*. The bacteria are then placed in a special medium of nutrients (culture) where they divide and thus multiple copies of each DNA fragment are produced (cloned).

The DNA fragments are produced by the action of enzymes which cleave the DNA of the organism at specific sites. Other enzymes then cause these fragments to become attached to the DNA of the vector. The vectors may be plasmids or bacteriophages. Plasmids are small circular pieces of DNA found in bacteria which render the bacteria which contain them resistant to various antibiotics. Bacteriophages are bacterial viruses which can penetrate the bacterial cell. The viral DNA then becomes integrated into the bacterial DNA and is reproduced along with it. These viruses can be rendered incapable of producing disease but still able to penetrate the bacterial cell so that their DNA becomes incorporated into the genetic apparatus of the bacterial cell.

Applications of recombinant DNA technology
The development of this technology involves potential blessings and fearful hazards to mankind.

The technique can be used for the identification of individuals who have abnormal genes which will cause them to suffer from a certain disease or to have children who will suffer from a disease. Scientists are at present attempting to isolate DNA fragments which contain, or are very close on the chromosome to, the genes for certain disorders. These fragments can then be rendered radioactive and used to identify those individuals in whom the gene of interest is likely to be abnormal. This method can be used for antenatal diagnosis by analysis of the DNA from amniotic fluid cells at

28

about 16-19 weeks of gestation. Alternatively a more recently introduced technique involving the sampling of chorionic villi can be used and defective genes in the fetus can be identified at 8-11 weeks of gestation. For example, DNA analysis has already been used in the antenatal diagnosis of haemophilia, Duchenne Muscular Dystrophy, sickle cell anaemia and cystic fibrosis. Another possibility is the analysis of DNA from blood cells for the identification of individuals with disorders before symptoms appear, or for the detection of individuals likely to have an affected child.

It is also possible, using this technique, to detect certain viruses in body tissues. For example, radioactive hepatitis B viral DNA has been used to demonstrate the presence of the virus in the liver and serum of some chronic hepatitis carriers.

Some biologically important substances can be synthesized by bacterial cells containing the appropriate human genes and these substances can be used in medical treatment. Two substances at present being produced in this way are insulin and human growth hormone. Vaccines are also being developed by this method *e.g.* for malaria.

It may be possible to use recombinant DNA technology for the treatment of genetic diseases in the not too distant future. However, such methods have formidable technical difficulties. For example in juvenile diabetes mellitus certain cells of the pancreas do not produce sufficient quantities of insulin. It has been suggested that a portion of these cells from a diabetic might be taken and grown in a cell culture medium. At the same time cells from healthy volunteers would also be grown and the gene that codes for insulin isolated from them. It might then be possible to introduce this genetic material into the cells of a patient in the culture medium and then to transfer these cells back into the pancreas of the patient where they would produce the necessary insulin.

However, it would be necessary to attach the normal gene to an inactivated virus in order to get it inside the diabetic person's cells. The viral DNA might not produce any ill effects in tissue culture but when transferred back into the patient's body it might do so. The cells containing the additional genetic material might be attacked and destroyed by the defence mechanisms of the body. It is even possible that the viral DNA might transform the cells into cancer cells.

A different approach to the treatment of genetic disease might be the injection of the normal gene into fertilised eggs. For example, a DNA fragment containing the gene for rat growth hormone was recently injected into fertilised mouse eggs and the mice which developed from these eggs grew much larger than their litter mates.[2]

Genetic engineering could also be applied to plants. Plants are unable to utilise nitrogen from the atmosphere (fix nitrogen) and have to obtain it from other substances e.g. fertilisers. But bacteria can fix nitrogen. If the genetic material that is responsible for nitrogen fixation in the bacteria could be placed directly into the plants the use of nitrogen-containing fertilisers would no longer be necessary.

Some plants are resistant to certain pests and diseases and others are not. Some genes which are responsible for such resistance have been identified and used to convert susceptible plants into resistant plants.

The human body is unable to synthesize all the amino acids necessary for the production of its proteins. People whose sole protein source is corn develop a deficiency disease called kwashikor because one of these amino acids is not produced by corn. If the gene responsible for the production of this amino acid could be transferred into corn plants these plants could be eaten as the sole source of protein without inducing a deficiency disease.

In a similar way it might be possible to introduce genes for desirable qualities into farm animals and improve milk or meat production.

2. R. D. Palmiter and others, 'Dramatic growth of mice that develop from eggs microinjected with metallothionein – growth hormone fusion genes', *Nature*, 1982; 300:611-5.

Possible hazards of recombinant DNA technology

Although there are many present and possible future benefits from genetic engineering, the potential hazards should
not be overlooked. The main fears have been of producing
organisms which contain, for example, genes causing susceptibility to cancer or genes which would render their bacterial host resistant to all known antibiotics. In the USA oil
eating micro-organisms are being developed to clear up oil
slicks but such an organism might go on to consume all
available oil.

Those who argue for the right to continue such experiments in spite of the hazards suggest that ultimately recombinant DNA will itself be a greater force for good than any
antibiotic or drug that humanity has ever known. According
to Emery[3] the consensus of scientific opinion now seems to
be that the dangers of these experiments have been much
exaggerated. Various authorities have laid down very careful
guidelines for research in this field including the construction
of special laboratories and the use of micro-organisms which
have been so treated that they cannot survive except in laboratory culture conditions. Nevertheless care will continue to
be necessary, for even in laboratories with special contain-
ment facilities infections are sometimes reported. Once a
modified bacterium has escaped there is no way to recall it.

In Vitro Fertilisation

In July 1978 the world's first so called 'test-tube baby' -
Louise Brown – was born. Dr Patrick Steptoe, a British gynaecologist, was able to obtain an unfertilised egg from the
baby's mother, fertilise it with her husband's sperm outside
her body, and after fertilisation place the embryo into her
womb. Since then several hundred babies have been born
after fertilisation outside the body.

The technique consists of first treating the mother with a
hormone which causes the ovary to produce several mature
ova. The ova are then removed by micro-surgery and mixed

3. Emery, *op. cit.*

with sperm in a petri dish. A few days after fertilisation the embryos have developed sufficiently to be inserted into the mother's womb.

Applications of in vitro *fertilisation*

The development of this technique has been welcomed as a means of allowing a certain group of infertile couples to have children of their own. In these couples, the fallopian tubes of the wife, where fertilisation normally takes place, are blocked and so it would be impossible for fertilisation to take place within the body. However, other questionable uses of this technique have at the same time been made a possibility. Some of these will be discussed below.

It may be possible in the not too distant future to separate the sperm producing male offspring from those which would produce female offspring. Thus couples could use this technique as a means of choosing the sex of their child. If couples were able to choose the sex of their children there might be an imbalance in the number of offspring of each sex produced. In many countries it is likely that more male offspring would be produced than female.

The ability to choose the sex of one's child would be very helpful to those couples for whom there is a risk that children of only one of the sexes may have a genetic disorder. For example, on average half the sons of a woman who is a carrier of the gene for haemophilia will be affected by this condition, whereas all her daughters will be normal. Therefore she could ensure having unaffected children by having only daughters.

Up to this point it has been assumed that the egg belongs to the woman herself and the sperm to her husband. However it is possible to fertilise the woman's egg with sperm from another man, and use the ovum of another woman and fertilise it with the husband's sperm. This could be useful when one or other partner is unable to produce ova or sperm. Alternatively, if one partner wishes to avoid passing on a genetic disorder to their children they may wish to use donated sperm or ova instead of their own.

In other cases a donated embryo might be used such that neither ovum nor sperm is from the woman or her husband. Related to this is the idea of the use of a surrogate mother whereby a woman can ask another woman to bear a child for her. The ovum and sperm producing the embryo can be from the donor woman and her husband or from the surrogate mother and the donor woman's husband.

In vitro fertilisation makes it possible for experiments to be carried out on human embryos. It has been suggested, for example, that in the future it might be possible to split an embryo at an early stage of development and several identical embryos (clones) would result. Experiments would then be carried out on some of the embryos to test for various defects and if these were not found one of the untested embryos would then be transferred to the woman's womb. The woman would then be assured that her child would be free from these defects. On the other hand, if defects were found in the embryos they would either be discarded or genetic engineering techniques such as those described earlier would perhaps be used to insert the missing gene into the embryo before it was implanted into the mother's womb.

The subject of experimentation on embryos is discussed in more detail elsewhere in this book.

It has also been suggested that in the future, clones might be produced by replacing the nucleus of a newly fertilised egg with the nucleus from a body cell. The new individual which then developed from the egg would have a genetic constitution identical to that of the donor of the body cell. Possibly people would produce clones of themselves specifically to act as organ donors. Since they would be genetically identical there would be no rejection problems in, for example, a heart and lung transplant. However this method of cloning is technically difficult and it would require much more research before it could become a practical possibility.[4]

---

4.   A. McLaren, 'Prenatal Diagnosis before Implantation: Opportunities and Problems', *Prenatal Diagnosis*, 1985, 5:85-90.

Another development of *in vitro* fertilisation might be the production of hybrids between humans and other species. At present, in the investigation of male sub-fertility, an attempt is made to fertilise hamster eggs with human sperm. In this test any resulting embryo does not develop beyond the two-cell stage. However, other forms of trans-species fertilisation tests might be developed which could result in embryos which would develop for a considerable period of time.

It has also been suggested that experiments might be attempted in which human embryos would be transferred to the uterus of another species for gestation.

Problems arising from the use of in vitro *fertilisation*

The advent of the possibility of *in vitro* fertilisation brings with it many ethical problems to which there are no easy solutions. Even in the simplest situation where a woman is carrying an embryo which is the product of her own ovum and her husband's sperm there is the possibility that the embryo might be damaged. The individual which developed from it might thus be handicapped. Would this individual or his parents be able to sue the scientist who carried out the *in vitro* fertilisation? At present there does not seem to be an increase in abnormalities among babies conceived in this way. However, there might possibly be a greater incidence among these individuals of conditions which are not obvious until adult life.

Another problem concerns the disposal of those embryos which are not required for implantation into the mother's womb. Usually several ova are taken from the woman and fertilised with the husband's sperm to ensure that at least one is suitable for implantation after fertilisation. Should the remaining embryos be destroyed? And if so does this constitute abortion? Is it right to freeze these embryos for possible implantation into the mother at a later date with the risk that they might become damaged by the process of freezing and thawing?

34

Even more problems arise when we consider the consequences of a woman carrying an embryo which is not entirely hers and her husband's. Consider, for example, the situation when a woman's ovum is fertilised by sperm which is not her husband's - either because he is infertile or for some other reason but nevertheless with his consent. Is the child legitimate? As the law now stands such a child would be illegitimate and registration of the child as the child of the husband would be a criminal offence.

The husband's attitude to the child might change if it were found to be in any way unusual and he might reject the child. If the couple were eventually to become divorced could the husband claim the right to see the child? The wife might claim that the child was uniquely hers.

Suppose a woman agrees to be a surrogate mother and to have another couple's embryo implanted into her womb so that she can bear the child for them. She may later decide that she wishes to keep the child in her womb and there would be a dispute between herself and the couple. At present there are no legal guidelines as to whose the child is, though the tendency has been for the courts to decide in favour of the woman who gave birth to the child.

At present, cloning by replacing the nucleus of a fertilised egg by the nucleus of a body cell seems a remote possibility. However if the technical difficulties could be overcome the consequences are potentially horrific. People might wish to produce copies of themselves and hire a woman as a surrogate mother of their clone. Alternatively, a woman might wish to bear a child who is a copy of someone she admires such as an Olympic athlete or an Einstein.

A further development from *in vitro* fertilisation is the idea of growing a baby from conception to term outside the body in an artificial environment. It has been suggested[5] that the next step will be to develop an artificial placenta so that

5. W. Walters, P. Singer (eds.), *Test Tube Babies, a Guide to Moral Questions, Present Techniques and Future Possibilities*, Oxford, 1983.

the embryos can develop until they are ready for incubators at about twenty-two weeks.

In July 1984 the Committee of Inquiry into Human Fertilisation and Embryology, under the chairmanship of Dame Mary Warnock, issued their report.[6] Some of the recommendations of this committee which relate to the issues discussed in this chapter are given below.

1. A new statutory licensing authority be established to regulate both research and those infertility services which we have recommended should be subject to control.
2. The service of IVF should continue to be available subject to the same type of licensing and inspection as we have recommended with regard to the regulation of AID.
3. Egg donation be accepted as a recognised technique in the treatment of infertility subject to the same kind of licensing and controls as we have recommended for the regulation of AID and IVF.
4. The form of embryo donation involving donated semen and egg which are brought together *in vitro* be accepted as a treatment for infertility, subject to the same type of licensing and controls as we have recommended with regard to the regulation of AID, IVF and egg donation.
5. It should be accepted practice to offer donated gametes and embryos to those at risk of transmitting hereditary disorders.
6. The AID child should in law be treated as the legitimate child of its mother and her husband where they have both consented to the treatment.
7. The law should be changed so as to permit the husband to be registered as the father.

6. Department of Health and Social Security, *Report of the Committee of Inquiry into Human Fertilisation and Embryology*, London, HMSO, 1984.

8. Legislation should provide that when a child is born to a woman following donation of another's egg the woman giving birth should, for all purposes, be regarded in law as the mother of that child, and that the egg donor should have no rights or obligations in respect of the child.

9. The legislation proposed in '7' and '8' should cover children born following embryo donation.

10. Legislation should be introduced to render criminal the creation or the operation in the United Kingdom of agencies whose purposes include the recruitment of women for surrogate pregnancy or making arrangements for individuals or couples who wish to utilise the services of a carrying mother, such legislation should be wide enough to include both profit and non profit making organisations.

11. The clinical use of frozen embryos may continue to be developed under review by the licensing body.

12. Research conducted on human *in vitro* embryos and the handling of such embryos should be permitted only under licence.

13. No live human embryo derived from *in vitro* fertilisation, whether frozen or unfrozen, may be kept alive, if not transferred to a woman beyond fourteen days after fertilisation, nor may it be used as a research subject beyond fourteen days after fertilisation. This fourteen day period does not include any time during which the embryo may have been frozen.

14. There should be a maximum of ten years for the storage of embryos after which time the right to use or disposal should pass to the storage authority.

15. The licensing body be asked to consider the need for follow-up studies of children born as a result of the new techniques, including consideration of the need for a centrally maintained register of such births.

16. Where trans-species fertilisation is used as part of a recognised programme for alleviating infertility or in the assessment or diagnosis of subfertility it should

be subject to licence and that a condition of granting such a licence should be that the development of any resultant hybrid should be terminated at the two cell stage.

17. The placing of a human embryo in the uterus of another species for gestation should be a criminal offence.

The Christian Response to these Techniques

What then should be the Christian response to the advent of these new techniques? The basic problem would seem to be the sanctity of human life, a subject which is dealt with in another chapter. We would probably see nothing wrong in these techniques being applied to animals. The criterion we would then use would be the avoidance of cruelty, not the intrinsic value in the animal's life. The value of a human life is that man was created in the image of God and can enter into a personal relationship with him.

In Genesis 1:28 man is commanded to replenish the earth and subdue it and to have dominion over the living creatures. This is a delegated authority and we should oppose any research which does not agree with biblical principles. Some people would say that all genetic engineering is wrong, whereas others would say that it is our duty to do all we can for our fellow men. However, man is finite and can make catastrophic mistakes especially when not living in obedience to the Creator.

Some of the possible consequences of recombinant DNA technology are unquestionably of benefit to mankind. For example, the production of biologically important substances such as insulin or the treatment of disease by altering the diseased tissue of the body. The improvement of animals and plants for more efficient food production would be especially valuable in under-developed countries.

Other consequences of this technology are not however so desirable. The technique facilitates antenatal screening and many Christians would be unhappy about this. This subject is dealt with in another chapter. In addition to antenatal screening, it might be possible to screen adults to see if they carried 'undesirable' genes and, if they did, they might be pressurised not to have children. Has man the right to say that some characteristics are desirable and others are not? Whereas God may have given man the ability to reduce the incidence of certain diseases, he does not intend that man should be a race of super-beings. Only one perfect man has ever lived and he is Jesus Christ.

When considering the technique of *in vitro* fertilisation there are again potential benefits to mankind, but it would seem that there are far more undesirable possible consequences of its usage. It could be argued that if a woman who is unable to have a child because of blocked fallopian tubes wishes to make use of this technique to have her and her husband's child, the ethical problems are no greater than if she had an operation on another part of her body. However, there is always the possibility that the embryo so produced might be damaged or die. It does not seem right for man to take the risk of destroying a human life for the sake of allowing a childless couple to have their own children.

In vitro fertilisation circumvents the necessity for new life to be produced by the union of one man and one woman as one flesh (Genesis 2:24). An embryo can be produced by the union of an egg cell from any woman with a sperm from any man. Is it going too far to say that by using this technique man is attempting to take on God's role as Creator? Perhaps man has succumbed to Eve's temptation to 'be as God'.

The idea of producing hybrids between man and other species by this technique is abhorrent. The seriousness with which God would regard such experiments is perhaps indicated in Leviticus 20:15-16, which says that people who have sexual relations with animals should be put to death.

It has been suggested that man's desire to produce clones or copies of himself is related to his desire for immortality.[7] Man has always believed in two things - the fact

7. D. T. Gish, C. Wilson, *Manipulating Life: Where Does it Stop?* San Diego, California, 1981.

of a power beyond himself and of a life beyond the grave. When a man thinks of cloning there is a sense in which he is searching for that life beyond.

Some have gone so far as to suggest that the introduction of these techniques points to the end of time.[8] For example II Thessalonians 2 speaks of increasing lawlessness in the world before the return of our Lord. Man has paid the penalty for insisting on his own will in the Garden of Eden, at the time of the Flood and at the Tower of Babel. When men started to build the Tower of Babel, God said 'This they begin to do and now nothing will be restrained from them, which they have imagined to do' (Gen. 11:6). Perhaps God is saying something similar today with regard to genetic engineering and *in vitro* fertilisation.

What man is seeking to achieve by these techniques God offers at the end of time to those who believe in Jesus.There will be a new heaven and a new earth, and there will be no more sickness, death, pain or sorrow. The nations will be healed by the leaves of the Tree of Life. That will include all the benefits of a human genetic system so restored to its original perfection that sickness and deformity will be eliminated.

8.   Gish and Wilson, *op. cit.*

MAN AS EXPERIMENTAL SUBJECT: EMBRYO RESEARCH AND ITS CONTEXT

Nigel M. de S. Cameron

The development of *in vitro* fertilisation and the associated revolution in reproductive medicine[1] led to the publication in 1984 of the Report of the Warnock Committee, charged with reporting to Her Majesty's Government on advances in 'human fertilisation and embryology'. Chief, and most contentious, among the matters on which Warnock had to report was whether, and if so in what circumstances, the early human embryo – available now to medical scientists in the laboratory as it had never been before – should be the subject of deleterious experimentation. The Committee recommended that experimentation should indeed be permitted on the embryo *in vitro*, up to 14 days after fertilisation.

In fact, such experimental use of the embryo had been current for a decade before Warnock reported, and necessarily lay behind the clinical development of human IVF. According to Warnock, it had not hitherto been possible to sustain an embryo *in vitro* for longer than 14 days. The Committee proposed a statutory licensing authority to supervise future embryo research, and as this essay goes to press it is anticipated that legislation will (finally) b e brought forward to enact the major Warnock proposals, although uncertainty remains whether a Parliamentary majority can be found to support legislative recognition for this central recommendation, and H. M. Government has indicated that a free vote will be allowed between alternative clauses on this issue.

Warnock considered two separate possibilities in respect of embryo research. In one case, research might be carried out on so-called 'spare' embryos, the by-product of the use of IVF to circumvent infertility. Three members of the Com-

1. Dr Susan Holloway has chronicled some of these developments in her essay elsewhere in this symposium.

mittee dissented from this recommendation. In another, ova might be fertilised specifically for experimental purposes. A further four members dissented here, so that the major recommendation of the Committee was actually endorsed by the smallest possible majority of its members.

Human embryo research has proved a most controversial public and political question. Yet much of the medical-scientific establishment, in Britain and elsewhere, has supported this development. It has been argued (with some reason) that for a society which allows the abortion of the maturing fetus on (often) trivial grounds to object to the careful experimental use of the zygote is both illogical and hypocritical.[2] It can scarcely be denied that widespread public and professional acquiescence in social abortion has been a powerful contributor to the medico-moral background to Warnock. By the same token, the pro-abortion lobby has been active in defence of Warnock, since they rightly view any legal protection afforded to the early embryo as ultimately subversive of liberal abortion. There can be no doubt that post-1967 abortion practice in Britain has prepared the ground for embryo research, and a similar pattern may be traced in other countries where IVF technology has followed in the wake of liberal abortion practice.

While opposition to the use of the human embryo for purposes of deleterious research has largely come from those who regard the human embryo as a human person, it should be noted that the minority on the Warnock Committee who dissented from any experimental use of the embryo did not do so on that ground. Theirs was a more limited case, and it is certainly possible to argue strongly against the practice on one of two grounds which do not depend upon such a conclusion as to the character of the embryo. The *potential* character of the early embryo, as forerunner of the personal human being, is – it can be argued – itself sufficient

2. As has been pointed out, for example, by Sir John Peel, 'After the Embryo the Fetus?', in *Embryos and Ethics*, edited by the present writer, Edinburgh, 1987.

reason to grant it respect and protection. Alternatively, it can be argued that, if we are *uncertain* as to the actual character of the early embryo – whether, or in what sense, we may call it a personal being – then such uncertainty, in a matter of this gravity, counsels caution. Only were we firmly convinced that we were not dealing with 'one of us' in a morally significant sense could research be approved. We mention these two lines of argument because each should carry considerable weight with some who are untouched by the kind of argument we present in this chapter.

The general question of the ethics of research on human beings has been helpfully and recently surveyed by Dr Richard Higginson.[3] In the western medical tradition respect for the sanctity of life and the dignity of the individual have led to an historical consensus that seriously deleterious research should never be undertaken on human subjects. This position was most recently set out in documents framed after the end of the Second World War. The principles were restated by the World Medical Association because the War had witnessed the gravest abuse to which they had ever been subject, and to that abuse we shall shortly turn. But its flagrant character must not distract us from the fundamental analogy which connects all such abuse of human dignity. The Declaration of Helsinki, in reiterating the prohibition of involuntary and deleterious research, was not merely reacting to particularly gross violations of this principle. It was re-asserting the fundamental dignity of the human person. When the nauseating and especially depraved elements in the following accounts have been removed, one thing remains: that human beings have been used for purposes of experiment. That ties together the events recounted below, and supplies the theme of our discussion.

3. In his chapter 'The Ethics of Experimentation' in *Embryos and Ethics, op. cit.*

The Medical Holocaust

Modern times have witnessed one great exception to the conventional prohibition on the use of human beings as experimental subjects. In a way that has fascinated historians even as it has disgusted them, significant elements within the German medical profession departed radically from the prevailing Hippocratic consensus during the years before the War, and their adoption of Nazi principles as an alternative finally led to the use of concentration camp inmates in Germany and the occupied territories as candidates for human vivisection.[4]

As simply one among the many horrors of the Nazi regime this use of prisoners for medical-scientific research, though resulting in the 'medical trials' at Nuremburg at which some of its major perpetrators were brought to account, has been largely eclipsed in the public mind by the extermination policy itself on which these research programmes were parasitic. The availability of large numbers of human persons who were in any event candidates for death encouraged a significant number of German physicians to engage in the kind of research on human subjects which had been consistently repudiated by humane medical practice. As Richard L. Rubenstein notes in *The Cunning of History*, once the principle was accepted that they had no rights, the 'utilization' of prisoners 'as human guinea pigs in the Nazi medical experiments' made sense:

> From the point of view of pragmatic rationality, devoid of religious or moral sentimentality, human beings are often the most suitable subjects for medical experiments. Dogs, guinea pigs, and monkeys are only partially acceptable surrogates.[5]

4. It is less well-known that prisoners-of-war held by the Japanese were also used for experimental purposes in camps in China, where biological warfare devices were apparently tested on inmates.
5. Richard L. Rubenstein, *The Cunning of History. Mass Death and the American Future*, New York, 1974, p. 48.

It was therefore not surprising that, in a society in which the prisoners – Jews and others – were not held to have the status and dignity of full human persons, they were rapidly subject to exploitation. Rubenstein continues:

> Once German physicians realized that they had an almost limitless supply of human beings at their disposal for experiments, some very respectable professors at medical schools and research institutes seized the unique opportunity. Their findings were reported at meetings of medical societies. On no occasion was any protest recorded.[6]

It is important to note that this treatment stemmed, as Rubenstein points out, from the perception that the Jews (and others) did not possess human dignity. Their treatment depended in an important measure not simply on their availability (and the lack of legal protection which, in practical terms, was its cause), but also on the general perception of them as non-persons. It is only possible to begin to account for the way in which the prisoners were treated overall – and not simply their medical abuse – by realising that their captors and doctors, many of them cultivated and compassionate men and women, did not *see* them as human persons. This is scarcely a defence of what was done, but it is a partial explanation of how it could have been done. By the same token, it serves as a partial explanation of how more recent abuses have been carried on in the name of medicine. A fundamental failure in imagination, a distortion in the perception of reality, lies at the root of the grossest of ethical distortions which followed. Only thus can these, and later, medical abuses be understood.

The story has been told in a number of places, but was classically brought before medical opinion in the post-War years by Dr Leo Alexander, an American psychiatrist who had been seconded to the War Crimes Commission at Nuremburg, in an article entitled 'Medical Science under

6. *Ibid.*, pp. 48f.

Dictatorship' published in the *New England Journal of Medicine* in 1949, and recently reprinted in *Ethics and Medicine*.

Alexander is anxious to set the medical experiments in the context of earlier developments in German medicine. Setting the scene, he writes as follows:

> Irrespective of other ideologic trappings, the guiding philosophic principle of recent dictatorships, including that of the Nazis, has been Hegelian in that what has been considered 'rational utility' and corresponding doctrine and planning has replaced moral, ethical and religious values. Nazi propaganda was highly effective in perverting public opinion and public conscience, in a remarkably short time. In the medical profession this expressed itself in a rapid decline in standards of professional ethics.

Alexander then surveys the medical developments which lay behind the abuses in the camps, and which prepared the way for them. He draws attention to the dramatic abandonment of the Hippocratic consensus in pre-War Germany, partly under the influence of the Nazi ideology, though in some degree preceding it. The period before the War saw the beginnings of a euthanasia programme within Germany which reflected a shifting pattern of ethical opinion. 'By 1936', Alexander can write, 'extermination of the physically or socially unfit was so openly accepted that its practice was mentioned incidentally in an article published in an official German medical journal.' In 1939 Hitler issued a first direct order for euthanasia, and a department was established to carry it through. Questionnaires were issued to state institutions about their long-stay patients, and ultimately 275,000 people, including many children, were exterminated. Alexander notes that those killed included 'the mentally defective, psychotics (particularly schizophrenics), epileptics and patients suffering from . . . infantile paralysis, Parkinsonism, multiple sclerosis and brain tumours.' 'Here', he writes, 'one sees what "euthanasia" means in actual practice.'

It is important to note these developments within Germany and before and during the early part of the War, since it

46

would otherwise be possible to dismiss the story of medicine under the Third Reich as a distortion brought about by war itself. On the contrary, it has been argued that the brutalisation of the extermination programme and the medical abuses associated with it were possible only because the ground had been cleared before ever the War began, in ethical discussion and, finally, in the euthanasia programme, within Germany itself – and within the German medical profession.

Alexander sums up the involvement of the German doctors in this way:

> Medical science in Nazi Germany collaborated . . . particularly in the following enterprises: the mass extermination of the chronically sick in the interest of saving 'useless' expenses to the community as a whole; the mass extermination of those considered socially disturbing or racially and ideologically unwanted; the individual, inconspicuous extermination of those considered disloyal within the ruling group; and the ruthless use of 'human experimental material' for medico-military research.[7]

Turning then to the abuse of prisoners, Alexander gives a series of harrowing instances of the research programmes undertaken in the concentration camps.

> One of the most revolting experiments was the testing of sulfonamides against gas-gangrene by Professor Gebhardt and his collaborators, for which young women captured from the Polish Resistance Movement served as subjects. Necrosis was produced in a muscle of the leg by ligation and the wound was infected with various types of gas-gangrene bacilli; frequently, dirt, pieces of wood and glass splinters were added to the wound. Some of these victims died, and others sustained severe mutilating deformities of the leg.[8]

To take a further example:

7. *New England Journal of Medicine*, July 14, 1949, p. 39. This important article is now available reprinted in *Ethics and Medicine* 3:3 (1987).
8. *Ibid.*, p. 44.

Live dissections were a feature of another experimental study designed to show the effects of explosive decompression. A mobile decompression chamber was used. It was found that when subjects were made to descend from altitudes of 40,000 to 60,000 feet without oxygen, severe symptoms of cerebral dysfunction occurred – at first convulsions, then unconsciousness in which the body was hanging limp and later, after wakening, temporary blindness, paralysis or severe confusional twilight states. [Dr Sigmund] Rascher, who wanted to find out whether these symptoms were due to anoxic changes or to other causes, did what appeared to him the most simple thing: he placed the subjects of the experiment under water and dissected them while the heart was still beating, demonstrating air embolism in the blood vessels of the heart, liver, chest walls and brain.[9]

One could, indeed, cite many, many instances of this degrading experimental programme. It is no surprise that in the aftermath of the 'medical trials' the World Medical Association sought to re-assert its fundamental opposition to such practices.[10] The question which arises is whether there is any relevant analogy between this deviant medical tradition and the subject of this chapter. Before we address that question we turn to consider another deviant narrative of experimentation. It brings us much closer to the specific question of research on human embryos.

9. *Ibid.*, pp. 42f.
10. The principles of the Hippocratic Oath were re-iterated by the World Medical Association in the Declaration of Geneva of 1949. In 1962 the WMA adopted the Declaration of Helsinki in which a series of principles for the experimental use of human subjects was laid down. In particular, we read that 'it is the duty of the doctor to remain the protector of the life and health of that person on whom the clinical research is being carried out'. It is interesting to note that one group formed to oppose the recommendations of the Warnock Committee, with the late Dr David Woollam, the distinguished Cambridge embryologist, as its first Chairman, has taken as its name the *Helsinki Medical Group* with the provisions of the Declaration of Helsinki as its point of departure in the defence of the human embryo.

Experiments on Live Fetuses

A second disturbing and unpleasant subject which we must review is that of the experimental use of the human fetus. When the Warnock Report first appeared and debate on the question of embryo research surfaced, the present writer in common with many others invoked the prospect of fetal experimentation as a hypothetical possibility which might follow on from the experimental use of the early embryo. In common with most people, he did not then realise that this was not science fiction, but science fact. Unknown to much informed opinion, the last thirty years and more have witnessed a stream of medical-scientific experiments upon human fetuses, experiments which have ended in the death of the fetus concerned.

No doubt there has been work which has been kept secret, or which has proved unproductive, and therefore never reached published form. But for those who know where to look there has been a series of published reports in the medical literature of live human fetuses, obtained after abortions, being kept alive so that experiments can be performed on them; and, subsequently, when their experimental value has ended, dying or being destroyed. We could look at any of a number of published examples.

For instance, in 1963 the *American Journal of Obstetrics and Gynecology* carried a report which began by describing the immersion of live fetal and new-born *mice* in a chamber of water at different pressures. It then continued without comment:

> Human fetuses in a closed chamber. During the first 30 minutes of immersion the temperature of the solution was raised from 15° to 30° C., and the oxygen pressure to 250 pounds per square inch. At intervals of 11 hours the chamber was decompressed gradually by dropping the pressure to one half the previous level every 10 minutes, until it was down at least to 15 pounds per square inch, before opening to see whether any animals had survived. Frequently, the umbilical cord was pulsating or heartbeats were visible; if not, the thorax was opened and the heart was observed directly. When the heart was beating, the fetus was returned to the chamber and the

experiment was resumed. The periods of survival of 15 human fetuses varying from 9 to 24 weeks of gestation are indicated in Fig. 2. No fetus was living after a third period of immersion of 11 hours.[11]

Since the prose of this chilling paragraph is not calculated to draw attention to the enormity of the experiment it describes, let us look at it again. Fetuses of between 9 and *24* weeks' gestation were subjected to immersion in a pressurised chamber for up to three periods of 11 hours each. At the end of each period the chamber was opened to see 'whether any animals had survived'. If no heartbeat was evident, 'the thorax was opened and the heart observed directly' to check. When the heart was still beating, the fetus was returned for a further period of 11 hours. After the third such period, they had all died.

Lest it be thought that work of this kind has been done only in America, we can look also at one of two papers published in the *Journal of Endocrinology* by M. C. Macnaughton and two separate collaborators (J. R. T. Coutts and Marion Greig) in the late 1960s. The second paper is entitled 'The Metabolism of [4-14C] Cholesterol in the Pre-Viable Human Foetus', and the aim of the research is reported as follows:

The experiments reported in this paper were carried out to determine whether the mid-term human foetus metabolizes cholesterol to progesterone. Solomon, Bird, Ling, Iwamiya & Young (1967) have published preliminary results which suggest that the mid-term foetus is unable to do so.[12]

The experiments were conducted upon 'foetuses of 13-22 weeks gestational age . . . obtained at therapeutic termina-

11. Robert C. Goodlin, 'Cutaneous Respiration in a Fetal Incubator', *American Journal of Obstetrics and Gynecology*, July 1, 1963, p. 574.
12. J. R. T. Coutts and M. C. Macnaughton, *Journal of Endocrinology* 44, 1969, p. 481.

tions of pregnancy'. The larger group of fetuses was treated as follows:

> Six foetuses were perfused by a modification of the method of Westin, Nyberg & Enhorning (1958). The foeto-placental unit was removed at laparotomy, the foetus separated and the umbilical vessels cannulated. The foetus was then immersed in 50% Hartmann's soln . . . in a closed system perfusion tank with a manometer to measure pressure changes caused by increase or decrease of blood vol. The blood was dripped into the umbilical vein and perfused through the foetus with the foetal heart acting as pump . . . . The perfused blood was collected from the umbilical artery. [4-^{14}C]Cholesterol . . . was injected into the umbilical vein and perfusion allowed to continue for 1 hr. at room temperature for four of the foetuses (gestational age 16-19 weeks) and for 2 hr. for the remaining two (gestational age 20-22 weeks). After perfusion, the foetus was dissected immediately, the organs removed, weighed and stored at - 20° until extracted . . . . After homogenization in a 'Virtis 23' (Exal Ltd.) high speed homogenizer (large organs) or grinding with sand in a mortar and pestle (small organs) . . . .[13]

13. *Ibid.*, p. 482.
Compare statements quoted in Alexander, *art. cit.*, with the following in defence of Warnock and embryo research from Professor M. C. Macnaughton, President of the Royal College of Obstetricians and Gynaecologists: 'Prevention of a serious condition is far better than waiting for it to occur and then giving treatment. This is done in embryo research and should it continue it may be possible to forecast and prevent such conditions as Down's Syndrome, Cystic Fibrosis or Muscular Dystrophy which are all very serious handicapping conditions . . . . Those who would deny the possibility of preventing these terrible handicaps must bear a heavy responsibility if the recommendation of the Warnock Committee on embryo research up to 14 days is banned [*sic*].' *The Times*, 1st December 1984. Macnaughton dismisses those who disagree as holding 'particular moral and religious views' as if this somehow condemned them, and as if he and those who agreed with him did not! It should be noted that this is the same Macnaughton who in the 1960s was involved in research on live fetuses, as indicated above.

Again, the effect of the scientific prose is to treat what is described as if it were somehow a normal, indeed typical piece of research. Yet its subject is a human being, and in two cases at least, a human being on the verge of viability.

It is true that many members of the medical profession would wish to disavow experimental work of this kind. But reputable journals have carried these reports, and experimenters have included distinguished members of the profession, one of whom sat on the Warnock Committee itself. These are facts of which the public should be aware, especially as it is repeatedly assured that the 14-day limit on embryo research would not be breached, and that a firm distinction can be made between those (early) embryos who may be the subject of experimentation, and later which may not.

The context of experimentation on the human fetus is plainly provided by liberal abortion. It is certainly no accident that the two British papers by M. C. Macnaughton and collaborators were published in the late 1960s, at the very time when the law on abortion was being liberalised. That liberalisation both made fetuses more widely available and, more important, marked a change in the public (and medical) perception of the fetus. It was a shift from the older view in which a fetus was almost invariably a child who would in due time be born, to the new view in which it was a matter of maternal and medical opinion *whether* the fetus would ultimately be born as a child, or whether the fetus would rather be aborted. There can be no doubt that this growing change in social attitudes during the 1960s, finally crystallised in the law of 1967, enabled doctors (and, to a lesser degree, mothers) to 'see' the fetus in a new way. It was only because they could so visualise the fetus that they could come to terms with – indeed, in so many cases could welcome – the practice of liberal abortion. Liberal abortion demands, and depends upon, the failure of doctor and mother alike to grasp what it entails; or, rather, to grasp that the being whose life is taken is in fact a human being – identical in character to the fetal human being carried by the woman who 'wants' her pregnancy to culminate in childbirth.

In a manner which has unmistakable parallels with what went on under the Third Reich, the actions and attitudes of those involved in abortion are explicable only on the assumption of a fundamental failure in imagination. They do not grasp the significance of what they are doing. If they did, they – or most of them – would not, could not, do it. It is only because they believe themselves to be doing something other than in fact they are, that they can. They perceive the fetus as less than a human being, and therefore they treat him or her as such. So compassionate and diligent doctors, and loving and gentle mothers, consent in the destruction of the children committed to their care.

And in that context – in a context in which imagination has failed to lay hold upon reality, and has grasped only an unreal *chimera* in its place – in that context alone we can explain and begin to understand the mentality of the fetal experimenter, as the man or woman whose conscience has been numbed and distorted by the false vision of human fetal existence which is implicit in the acceptance of the disposability of fetal life implicit in abortion.

The Ethics of the Embryo
And so it is with embryo research.[14] It is possible only in a society which has long come to terms with liberal abortion, even though it may have drawn back (temporarily, at least) from the use of the live human products of abortion for experimentation themselves. We have already pointed out that, from the perspective of logic, for a society which allows

14. These issues are explored at greater length in *Embryos and Ethics. The Warnock Report in Debate*, edited by the present writer, Edinburgh, 1987. In his introductory chapter he outlines the distinctively Christian case against the view of the embryo implicit in Warnock, namely that in the incarnation of the Son of God the personal life of God himself was incarnated in the product of human conception.

abortion to baulk at embryo research is seemingly unreasonable. This need not in fact be so, for (it could be argued) experimentation is one step further along the road of disrespect from killing itself. But the connection is not chiefly in logic, it is – as we have suggested in another context – in imagination. Two men who are humane and compassionate face the issue together. To one, deleterious research on the embryo is an evil of incomprehensible proportions. To the other, it is the prudent use of medical-scientific technique to investigate and alleviate disease. To one, it involves the vile defacement of a human person who bears the image of God himself and who has a destiny in eternal glory. To the other, it involves the respectful use of 'human material' of no more significance than the sperm or ovum out of which it has come. These differences in perception are as fundamental as they could be. The single object of perception – the human embryo – is 'seen' by two different men as two wholly distinct entities. It is no surprise that in this debate there is little meeting of minds.

But what *is* the human embryo? The Christian's response is here distinctive, although – curiously – there are Christians who would not share it; and it rests on grounds which are open to those who are not. The human embryo, none would doubt, is a human being, a member of the species *Homo sapiens*, a fellow-member of the biological race with us. The fundamental question is: does this answer the ethical question, or does it not? Is our ethical notion of who is a human being to be governed by the realities of biology and genetics, or by something else? That is, do we (as societies, as legislators and jurists, as doctors) – do we have a right to impose our own categories of humanness upon the reality which we confront, or must we permit that reality to impress itself upon us and determine the categories in which we shall understand it?

There are distinctively Christian elements in such an argument, since Holy Scripture gives its own evidence as to the character of unborn human life, and the species-specific nature of the *imago Dei*. But Christian and non-Christian

54

alike are confronted by the need to choose between an ethical system which arises from reality and one which is imposed (as we choose) upon it. It is only by means of the latter that embryo research can find justification.

And here we find the fundamental significance of the harrowing accounts which we have cited above. For all their wide disparity, they are instances of a single principle: the use of human subjects for deleterious experimentation. So it is with research on the early embryo. And while the Nuremburg medical trials revealed a uniquely evil catalogue of conduct, and the narratives of fetal experimentation on the verge of viability are doubtless more shocking than those of early embryo research, the principle remains the same: human beings used as experimental objects, and in a way that is possible only because of a massive failure in imagination by those who conceive and perpetrate such acts. Of course, there are men who could use their own kind in this way and face the monstrous ethical implications of so doing. But most men could not, and do so – if they do so – only by divorcing their action from its roots in reality, and grasping with their imagination something other than is the case. It is a tragedy that good men, or men who were once good, should so be deceived by a warping of their perception, and though it does not alter the character of their actions, it is an essential element in their explanation. But it does not lessen what is done, or alter its profoundly evil character. For man's abuse of his own kind for experimental purposes must rank as the most dreadful of all his abuses of himself. The disinterested character of (some of) those involved, far from lessening and justifying what they do, serves to heighten its significance by underlining the degradation to which man is putting his fellow, treating as a mere laboratory artefact one who bears the divine image. Yet it is also, perhaps, a ground of final forgiveness: they know not what they do.

ANTENATAL SCREENING: BIBLICAL AND PASTORAL CONSIDERATIONS

David J. C. Easton

Introduction

The progress of medical technology poses many new problems for theology and ethics. In the absence of any clear directives from Scripture or guidance from Christian tradition, the Christian has to apply general biblical principles to situations for which there is no precedent. It is not surprising, therefore, that in untried ethical situations, the conclusions reached are often tentative and the solutions offered open to debate. The development of antenatal screening is a case in point.

The term 'screening' implies that a whole population is surveyed, with the aim of picking up a particular problem. Antenatal care, whilst now accepted as a normal part of having a baby, is a quite recent phenomenon (developed over the last 50 years). The first challenge was to reduce maternal deaths and later on to reduce perinatal deaths (stillbirths plus newborn losses). Because great strides have been made in achieving the present low figures, there is a relatively small residue of babies affected during pregnancy by 'avoidable' or 'unavoidable' factors.

Infections, such as syphilis in the mother, may affect the baby to a greater or lesser degree; up until the present day in many obstetric units, one of the routine blood tests performed on 'booking' at the antenatal clinic checks for this. Other blood tests investigate the rhesus factor, immunity to German measles and so on. In areas of high immigrant population, conditions such as sickle-cell anaemia (occurring in those of neg. 0 descent) are sought and may be treated during pregnancy. Ultrasound scanning has probably been the most dramatic advance in antenatal screening over the past couple of decades.

The selective abortion of malformed fetuses is a relatively new development and raises many theological and

56

ethical questions. Many who condemn abortion on demand feel that the abortion of the grossly handicapped is justified. It is an act of mercy; the parents are relieved of the burden of caring for a handicapped child; the welfare state is spared the cost of looking after such people. Thus selective abortion is defended on the grounds that it offers a ready solution to the human, social and economic cost of caring for the disabled. Some would go further and say that it is immoral and irresponsible knowingly to bring a handicapped child into the world. Antenatal screening is therefore seen as a technological blessing which should be welcomed - as reflected in the remark of a well-meaning Job's comforter to a mother who had just given birth to a spina bifida baby, 'What a pity you didn't have the test!' But the Christian looks beyond pragmatic considerations to the biblical, theological, and ethical principles which bear upon the issue. How ought we to handle the knowledge which antenatal screening provides? If the procedure is followed by abortion, do the arguments against abortion in general also apply to selective abortion? If, on the other hand, the antenatal diagnosis of handicap does not necessarily imply that the pregnancy should be terminated, what benefits does antenatal screening bring? Is screening for all a desirable goal?

Biblical Principles
The Mosaic law did not legislate for deliberately induced abortion, but the provision of Exodus 21:22 condemns the practice by implication. The New Testament has nothing to say about abortions as such, but there may be an allusion to it in Paul's mention of 'sorceries' (pharmakeia) among 'the works of the flesh' in Galatians 5:20, and in the references to sorcerers (pharmakoi) in Revelation 21:8 and 22:15. The 'pharmakoi' are literally 'mixers of potions', and in New Testament times these potions included abortifacient drugs.[1]

1. Gordon Wenham, 'Abortion: what about deformity before death?' *Third Way*, July/August 1981.

If the direct biblical evidence is less than specific, there are, however, other considerations which should be taken into account:

a. Scripture throughout upholds the sanctity of life and forbids the taking of human life except in the case of the convicted criminal (Gen. 9:6).
b. The Bible affirms that life begins at conception. This presupposition lies behind the stories concerning the birth of Esau and Jacob (Gen. 25:23), Samson (Jud. 13:7), John the Baptist and Jesus (Lk. 1:15 and Matt. 1:20).

The question, 'When does life begin?', is at the heart of the abortion debate. Several thresholds have been distinguished in the progress of the sperm-ovum-fetus development. There are those who regard the sperm as having human qualities. Contraception is therefore akin to homicide if not murder. This view is based on a misunderstanding of what happens at conception. Some argue that life begins when the sperm and the ovum unite, since from that moment a genetically unique being is created. Others draw the line at the point when the fertilised ovum attaches itself to the womb and begins to draw sustenance from the mother, or when the cerebral cells begin to grow at about forty days. Life is distinguished by the capacity to grow. Those of a more permissive outlook would aver that the fetus only acquires the right to exist as a human person at the point at which the mother begins to relate to the fetus as her baby; or at viability; or at birth itself.

What these differing standpoints share in common is an innate respect for life and humankind. Here a parallel may be drawn with the respect paid to a human corpse, whose dignity is safeguarded by law. It is no longer human as the fertilised ovum is not yet human. Yet there is the recognition that in some sense it is more than a collection of tissue. The point is illustrated by the replies two moral theologians, one of them a Roman Catholic and the other Anglican gave to the question. Faced with a test-tube containing a fertilised human egg surplus to requirements, what would they do? The Roman Catholic said he would put it on one side until he was sure that it was dead and then pour it respectfully down the sink. The Anglican said he would pour it down the sink straightaway, respectfully.[2]

c. Scripture teaches that the embryo is God's work and that the development of the fetus is the object of his care (Ps. 139:13-16, Eccles. 11:5, Is. 49:1) God sees future potential in the first beginnings of life.

d. Even the handicapped are not outwith God's sovereign will and purpose (Ex. 4:11). He has a special concern for the handicapped (Lev. 19:14 and Deut. 27:18). To deny the handicapped the possibility of life is to violate the spirit of God's law.

e. The imitation of God in Christ in our relationships with one another is a recurring theme in the ethical teaching of the New Testament. Thus in marriage the husband plays the role of Christ and the wife that of the church. Similarly, in the home parents take the place of God, and love and discipline their children as God the Father loves and disciplines his family, the church. It follows that when parents consent to abortion, they are departing from the divine pattern of parental love. The imitation of Christ is particularly relevant in determining the conduct of the Christian doctor. Christ is the Great Physician, the healer of all physical and spiritual ills. To the Christian doctor we must put the question: Is the practice of abortion compatible with that pattern of healing which we see in the ministry of our Lord?[3]

The teaching of Scripture is clear. The fetus is a life which God has created in his image, and for which he has a care, even if it suffers from deformity. The biblical principles which

2. Quoted by Clifford Longley, 'Question of Embryos from a Christian Point of View', *The Times*, September 30, 1982.
3. Gordon Wenham, *op. cit.*

have traditionally guided the Christian conscience in relation to abortion apply also to the selective abortion of the deformed.

The *Abortion Act* of 1967 allows abortion when two registered doctors believe in good faith 'that there is a substantial risk that if the child were born it would suffer from such physical and mental abnormalities as to be seriously handicapped'. We shall come to the ethical problems inherent in abortion on the grounds of some actual or potential defect. A legitimate distinction may be drawn between a fetus as grossly deformed (where, for instance, no brain has formed, or where the malformation is such that, if born, it could not possibly survive) and a fetus with a deformity not incompatible with life (as in the case of mongolism). In the first case it is arguable that abortion is justified, but in the second it is hard to see what difference exists between intentionally letting a mongol die after birth and aborting the fetus before birth. If the one is condemned as infanticide, how can the other be morally acceptable? Antenatal screening must be judged an accessory before the fact.

Ethical Considerations

Until recently, antenatal screening was only offered to women who, for one reason or another, were thought to be at risk of giving birth to a handicapped child, either because of some chromosomal or genetic defect in one or both parents, or because the mother had already given birth to a handicapped child (the chances of having a second child with spina bifida are one in four) or because she was over forty, when the risk of bearing a mongol is twenty times greater than in the case of a woman of twenty-five. Such women have usually thought carefully about their situation and the possible outcome of a pregnancy. The dilemma of whether or not to have an abortion, if tests indicate that the fetus is malformed, will in most cases have been faced beforehand.

The trend now, however, is to make antenatal screening more generally available. Between July 1976 and June 1977 half of the 22,000 women attending antenatal clinics in the

60

Glasgow area agreed to give specimens of blood for screening tests at sixteen to twenty weeks. Of the 11,585 women tested only 196 showed a raised concentration of alpha protein. Further checking of other factors which might have caused the raised value showed that 121 were false positives. Of the remaining 75 women, all but two agreed to amniocentesis. Tests of the amniotic fluid found evidence of fetal abnormality in 34 cases, and all but one of these pregnancies were terminated. All the aborted fetuses had major abnormalities.[4]

This trend towards screening for all is opposed by some in the medical profession on the grounds, first, of safety, and then of reliability. Amniocentesis is not without risk. But the reliability of the procedure also causes misgivings. The test is claimed to be 99 per cent reliable, and the results of the screening project in Glasgow bear that out. However, even a margin of error of 0.02 per cent means that one in every 500 aborted fetuses will be normal. G. R. Dunstan states that apart from some conditions like chromosomal disorders or enzyme deficiencies which can be diagnosed positively by amniocentesis, 'the most that can be predicted is a statistical risk of defect – as high as 50% for rare conditions, e.g. haemophilia (if the fetus is male), but much lower for other disorders, such as those arising from maternal contact with rubella. To terminate on the basis of statistical risk is to accept the necessity of killing more healthy fetuses than defective ones.'[5]

For many in the medical profession such a risk is ethically unacceptable. Even when abnormality is positively diagnosed, there remains the question of the nature of the handicap (what sort of defects justify abortion?) and the degree of handicap (is the defect treatable or incompatible with life?). In a day when normal fetuses are aborted on demand, the case for an abortion where an abnormality has been diagnosed is all too often looked on as compelling, without re-

4. See *The Lancet*, June 24th, 1978.
5. G. R. Dunstan, *The Artifice of Ethics*, London, 1974, p. 85.

gard for either the nature or the degree of handicap. The advent of screening for all would exert strong social pressures on women to undergo the test, even if they did not wish to.

Professor John Lorber of Sheffield, who is an acknowledged authority on the treatment of spina bifida, and who considers it not only permissible but essential to have an antenatal screening programme, tries to put the whole matter in perspective:

> Out of every 100 pregnancies in high risk families, only five will be affected by neural tube defects; two of these will have anencephaly and would not result in a viable child; one will have mild spina bifida, not diagnosable by alpha-fetoprotein tests, and only two will have large open spina bifida which can be diagnosed, and followed by termination, if the mother attends early enough for this to be carried out and if she agrees. So, out of 100 only two potentially viable babies would be aborted and one of those is likely to die early in life, even if fully treated . . . . Termination of pregnancy is legal on very many grounds, and well over 100,000 pregnancies are terminated every year in Britain alone of which the overwhelming majority of fetuses are normal. How does this compare with a few hundred terminations in which the fetus is abnormal?[6]

The question which concerns many, however, is the consequences of an explosion of antenatal screening on society. Since the *Abortion Act* of 1967 over two million pregnancies have been terminated. The result has been a dramatic increase in our tolerance of abortion. The coming years could see a similar change in our attitudes to prenatal abnormalities. Though Lorber says that 'no one in any civilised society should attempt to make such tests, or the termination to follow, compulsory', women who do not undergo screening could feel that they were acting irresponsibly. Those who do may be faced with the decision whether or not to terminate the pregnancy. In the nature of the case, the decision has to be taken quickly. Will hard-pressed obstetricians have the

6. 'A Question of Ethics', *Link* (published by the Association for Spina Bifida and Hydrocephalus) May/June 1980, p. 3.

time and patience to discuss the possibilities with the parents? In the present moral climate there will be an inclination towards abortion, whatever the nature or degree of the handicap. The elimination of the malformed could well colour society's attitude towards the handicapped who are born because of their parents' opposition to abortion and encourage the view that such children should not have been born. If that sounds far-fetched, the case of the doctor who jabbed the legs of a newly born spina bifida baby with a needle and then turned to the mother who had refused termination, and said, 'Spina bifida. But then, of course, you knew', before turning his back on her and walking away, illustrates the danger of intolerance and also how easily the dignity and worth of the handicapped can be demeaned. They could soon be seen as a needless and unwelcome burden on society and the state. In consequence, we would become an even less caring and humane society than we at present are.

Admittedly the abortion of the handicapped is often justified on the grounds of humanity and compassion. Lorber charges those who knowingly encourage the birth of severely handicapped infants with irresponsibility and inhumanity; and from a Christian standpoint, Professor Kalland asks, 'Are we sure, on biblical grounds, that it is always the just and loving thing to bring into this demanding, complex world a badly deformed, perhaps even mentally incomplete individual? While the scriptures establish the sanctity of life, the stress of scripture is on the quality of life.'[7]

The dilemma for doctors and parents can be acute. However, the argument from compassion requires close scrutiny for the following reasons:

a. May the argument from compassion not obscure the real motive for aborting a handicapped fetus, namely, the simple, quick, and efficient disposal of a problem? Abortion is more often a solution to a problem than an

7. Quoted by Richard Winter, 'Abortion – the Continuing Ambivalence', *Third Way*, July/August 1982.

act of mercy. In considering abortion, parents must scrutinise their motives rigorously.

b. If the abortion of a fetus on compassionate grounds is justified, then by the same argument the infanticide of the handicapped child or euthanasia may be justified.

Antenatal screening raises complex ethical problems for both doctors and parents. Only those who have no moral qualms about eliminating the handicapped by abortion will press for antenatal screening for all, since the procedure has limited value unless the diagnosis of handicap is followed by termination. Those who believe that abortion in general is wrong and that the selective abortion of the handicapped is only rarely justified, will not favour the extension of screening procedures. It confronts parents with a choice which in most cases they are ill-prepared to make. It assumes that living with handicap is a wholly negative experience which must be avoided at all costs. Much is sometimes made of the views of handicapped people themselves who openly say that they wish they had not been born or had been allowed to die in infancy. It would be arrogant and insensitive to minimise the suffering, both physical and emotional, of those born with handicap or to overlook the stress which handicap causes the family. But the Christian sees life, even when limited by handicap, as a gift from God which ought to be valued. And while acknowledging pain and suffering as an inescapable aspect of human existence in a fallen world, he looks forward to the final redemption of this world when God will open the eyes of the blind, the lame shall leap, and the dumb sing for joy (Is. 35:5 and 6).

Pastoral Considerations
The dilemma which faces many pregnant women who are not in favour of abortion is whether or not to undergo antenatal screening. What is the point of the procedure if she is not willing to terminate the pregnancy should the child she is carrying be diagnosed as handicapped? The knowledge that

the pregnancy will culminate in the birth of a handicapped child will turn happy expectation into anxious dread. How can parents cope with such knowledge?

Of course, those who agree to have the pregnancy terminated also suffer. The price of abortion in terms of emotional upset, feelings of guilt, and marital tension is high. A survey carried out in America revealed that 92 per cent of mothers and 82 per cent of fathers suffered from depression after abortion on medical grounds, and that 31 per cent of married couples separated.[8] Dr Kenneth McAll, a surgeon and consultant psychiatrist, claims that in an eighteen month period he dealt with 200 families which were spiritually disturbed by abortion.[9] The counselling and care of such people must be a matter of concern to the church. But parents who cannot countenance abortion and are therefore hesitant to accept antenatal screening, also have claims on our compassion and help. For mothers at high risk, antenatal screening followed by termination offers the possibility of having a normal child. If they have already given birth to a handicapped child, they would not risk another pregnancy if there were no antenatal test. The choice is then between 1. screening followed by abortion if handicap is diagnosed, 2. the possibility of having another handicapped child, or 3. having no more children. If our understanding of the teaching of Scripture is correct, then the third option presents a responsible way of resolving the dilemma. But it is a hard choice and parents need counselling and support in arriving at their decision.

Some who are at risk wish to be screened in order that they may have time to prepare themselves emotionally and in other ways for the birth of a handicapped child. Not all could cope with such knowledge and would feel it better to await the outcome of the pregnancy, albeit in fear and hope. But those who choose to know need particular support. It is

8. Quoted by Gordon Wenham, *op. cit.*, from F. Fuchs, *Scientific American*, June 1980.
9. 'Abortion – the Spiritual Legacy', an interview with Dr Kenneth McAll, in *Third Way*, April 6, 1978.

not enough for Christians to be anti-abortionist. This will involve the church in caring for parents who have been told
that their child will suffer handicap, in preparing the family for
the arrival of a handicapped child, and in providing the
understanding and support which will carry them through the
crisis of the birth and beyond into the often physically and
emotionally demanding routine of caring for a handicapped
child. A concern for moral principle is no substitute for caring
action.

Women who are not in the risk category but are encouraged to undergo screening as a matter of routine only to be
told that the fetus is abnormal, also find themselves in a
dilemma. Very often the implications of the test have not
been fully explained to them, perhaps because the doctor
assumes that they understand. They have never thought
through the ethics of abortion. Suddenly they are faced with
the question of whether or not to terminate the pregnancy. A
decision must be reached within a few days. If the fetus is so
grossly deformed that the child would die at birth, the choice
may be straightforward. But where the diagnosis is less
clear-cut, or where a case of mongolism is detected, the
choice is not so simple. Given the permissive attitude of
many in the medical profession towards abortion, it is likely
that the mother-to-be will be advised to have an abortion,
whatever the prognosis. It would take a very principled
woman to go against her doctor's advice. There is therefore a
great need, in the context of the Christian congregation or
fellowship, to encourage people to think through the issues
involved biblically so that they do not suddenly find themselves confronted by a problem of which they are scarcely
aware.

In a wider context, Christians should be active in shaping
public attitudes towards abortion and handicap. The ability of
the family to cope with handicap will determine to a large
extent the quality of life the handicapped child will enjoy. The
parents' response to their child will, in turn, be influenced to
some extent by the prevailing social attitudes towards people who are handicapped. The elimination of handicap, as we

have already suggested, could create a society in which handicap is not tolerated. Christians will stand for the dignity and worth of all humankind. Since life begins with conception, the fetus also has its value, which is not diminished by abnormality.

Handicap is not a reason for disposal. Since antenatal screening is often followed by abortion, Christians cannot be happy with its indiscriminate use. In the words of a doctor at a meeting of the British Medical Association: 'No longer should doctors agree to the termination of one individual to ease the discomfort and social inconvenience of another; or even to ease what we perceive as the discomfort and suffering of the proposed victim.'

LIFE ISSUES (1): ABORTION

Pamela F. Sims

The term 'abortion' implies loss of a pregnancy at a stage too early to allow for survival of the organism. When this occurs in nature it is called a 'spontaneous' abortion, it may be 'complete' or 'incomplete', the womb retaining fragments of afterbirth. There is 'threatened' abortion where bleeding presents yet the pregnancy, thus far, is intact. A 'missed' abortion, on the other hand, means the fetus has died in the uterus without any outward visible sign. It is retained sometimes for many months in the natural state, though usually the uterus is emptied by medical or surgical methods. Interestingly, certain mammals, such as rabbits, regularly abort their pregnancies without any external evidence - by process of reabsorption, when conditions are not favourable for them to reproduce.

The word 'abortion' of recent years has come to take on a completely different connotation. We are living in the era of 'induced' abortion. A new vocabulary has sprung up to cope euphemistically with what is now one of the most commonly performed gynaecological operations in, dare we say, the *world* today.

'Therapeutic' abortion was the earliest term, still sometimes used when the operation is done for strictly medical reasons; in other words it is treatment. In the early days of easier abortion social indications were also included in this term. 'Termination of pregnancy' (TOP) is probably most commonly used these days, and 'products of conception' (POCs) are the contents of the pregnant uterus. We have even learned to salve our consciences in making up operating lists containing cases of 'cyesis' (pregnancy) for 'VAT' (Vacuum Aspiration Termination) or 'STOP' (Suction TOP) or even 'Matburn D & C (after one of the first suction machines).

It must be remembered that pregnancy may require 'termination' at a later stage, when the baby is capable of survival, for the mother or baby's sake. Further, the same drugs and surgical techniques may be used in obstetric and gynaecological practice generally; for instance the missed abortion is usually removed by vacuum aspiration.

Historically, abortion has always been available within the framework of the law to save the mother's life. Until 1967, abortion for any other indication was illegal. Estimates of the number of women having abortions prior to that date are open to speculation; only the ones going wrong or resulting in death would reach official records. Those lobbying for easier abortion, although misguided, hoped that an ease in the law would somehow overcome the great discrepancy that existed between rich and poor. It was believed that there was already safe abortion for the rich, though again there are no figures to prove this. It is unlikely that those responsible for seeing through the Act of Parliament passed in 1967, operational from 1968 onwards, could have envisaged the state of affairs today which amounts to 'abortion on demand'.

The 1967 Act is so loosely worded that many interpretations are possible. The health and well-being not only of the woman but the rest of her family, if threatened by the pregnancy, in the opinion of two registered medical practitioners, may now legally allow for termination of pregnancy. The other main arm of the Act permits abortion when there is a 'substantial risk' that the child will be born handicapped. The situation prevailing up and down the country is that each gynaecologist interprets the law as he sees fit in the light of his own conscience. In defence of the average practitioner, from the start he resented having this new law thrust upon him. Consultant gynaecologists, perhaps without having fully thought out the issues at stake, were swept along by the mood of the nation, and honestly believed they were offering some sort of service. Abortion is a nasty job that has to be done. Needless to say in the private sector (and note that around half the abortions performed in this country are non-NHS) are found some unscrupulous characters who have made their fortunes out of abortion, but these must be the exception rather than the rule.

The so-called 'conscience clause' of the 1967 Act allows medical staff to opt out of abortion operations. There have always been doctors who have refused to be involved, and rather interestingly there are signs that more recently some are becoming disillusioned with abortion. Noteworthy is Bernard Nathanson who stopped performing abortions after running one of the largest abortion clinics in the U.S.A. He described his experience in *Aborting America*[1]. Without any religious change of heart he methodically argues the case against abortion, on humanitarian grounds. In this country too there are those who for various reasons have stopped doing abortions, realising that abortion has not really solved anything.

Abortion solves the immediate 'problem' but the long-term effects, especially with regard to guilt feelings, are difficult to measure scientifically. On a national level the utopia promised by the pro-abortionists with 'every child a wanted child' simply has not materialised. Child abuse and baby battering persist, marriages break down more than ever, and teenage pregnancy increases dramatically. And women, far from being 'liberated', find themselves more than ever at the mercy of society when it comes to deciding the fate of their unborn child.

Abortion Methods

Various methods of abortion have evolved to terminate the pregnancy as safely as possible (for the mother) according to the period of gestation. This is normally counted, for convenience, in weeks from the date of the onset of the last menstrual period. Ovulation, the release of the egg (ovum) from the ovary, occurs about 12 to 14 days after that date. The egg is wafted down the fallopian tube towards the cavity of the womb (uterus) by a current caused by tiny hair cells lining the opening of the tube, and muscular contractions within its wall. Fertilization, that is the penetration of the egg cell by a single sperm (the first to get there!), takes place within

1. *Aborting America*, Bernard Nathanson, New York, 1979.

the fallopian tube. This may occur up to 72 hours after sexual intercourse. Once the egg cell has been penetrated its wall immediately becomes resistant to the entry of further sperm; the genetic material combines and cell division of this unique new being rapidly takes place. Twins develop either as a result of the fertilization of two separate eggs (non-identical), or the development of two separate individuals from one fertilized egg sometime after fertilization (these are genetically identical).

Within a few days a fluid-filled space has formed inside the ball of cells (now called 'blastocyst') and it is on its way into the womb's cavity. The process of implantation next occurs: the blastocyst must embed in the lining of the uterus if pregnancy is to continue as the developing cells soon require a more efficient method of gaining nourishment than simple absorption from the surrounding maternal fluids. Once implantation takes place the forerunner of the placenta forms.

The moment of fertilization signifies, from the genetic point of view, the creation of a new individual. The egg and the sperm are not complete human cells in that they contain only half the normal complement of 46 chromosomes. During their development, before the penultimate division of the germ cell, they in fact contain twice the normal number of chromosomes. This phase allows the opportunity for the genetic material to mix; it is then randomly distributed in the subsequent divisions; this results in 23 chromosomes each in the final egg and sperm cell. In the case of the egg cell, this division is very unequal. One half keeps all the cell matter and the now surplus genetic material is extruded as a 'polar body'. When this has occurred twice, the nucleus occupies a relatively large cell. This is important as the cell matter provides material which will be utilised by the new cells formed by the fertilized egg.

Under natural conditions the egg and sperm cells cannot develop any further. Of interest are certain lower animals who can produce new offspring through fertilization of the egg by its own polar body. Some have proposed this explanation for 'immaculate' conception in man, and suggest that

71

Christ may have been conceived in such a manner. This idea is immediately quashed by pointing out that all the offspring of such a union would automatically be female (the combination of the two X chromosomes produced by division of the normal female XX containing cells)!

Interception Methods of Abortion
In this country the most commonly used methods of interrupting a pregnancy during its very early days are the intrauterine (contraceptive) device (IUD or IUCD) and to a lesser extent the progestagen-only pill (also known as the 'mini-pill'). IUDs are made of plastic and many contain copper. The mechanism of their action is still not completely understood. The principal effect is that the endometrium, the lining of the womb, is rendered hostile to the blastocyst, preventing implantation. Furthermore, tubal motility may be altered so that there is a slowing of the passage of the developing egg cells into the uterus. This would explain the higher incidence of ectopic pregnancy (a pregnancy developing outside the womb) known to occur in IUD users. Copper-containing devices may also exert a direct effect on the sperm themselves, preventing them from reaching the egg.

The progestagen-only type contraceptive pill is not to be confused with the modern, low dose, 'combined' pill. The latter contains a mixture of the female hormones, oestrogen and a progestagen, a synthetic version of the naturally occurring hormone, progesterone. The dose of hormone in the mini-pill is very low, but it exerts a contraceptive effect through a variety of mechanisms, similar to those described above. Under the influence of progesterone the mucus become thick and hostile to sperm. Should any manage to make the journey through the uterus to fertilize an egg, tubal motility is affected and the endometrium rendered unfavourable. The rate of ectopic pregnancy is also high in women who become pregnant on the progestagen-only pill.

The use of the 'morning after' pill was controversial as the general public first became aware of its use - how quickly we became accustomed to it. The ordinary combined contraceptive pill is given in larger than normal dosage, within 72 hours of unprotected sexual intercourse and will prevent pregnancy by causing a possibly fertilized egg to pass out of the uterus without implanting. Similarly, a copper IUD may be inserted up to 7 days after unprotected intercourse. The arguments surrounding those post-coital means of 'contraception' were, in the eyes of many, rather illogical. If the IUD is acceptable to prevent pregnancy, why should there be such a fuss about using these same means *after* intercourse, when it functions in exactly the same manner? The *Offences Against the Person Act*, 1861, however, states that it is the *intent* to procure an abortion that is illegal, whether or not the woman is indeed pregnant. The intention of the operator when he deliberately inserts a coil (or prescribes pills) post-coitally is arguably distinct from that of the doctor supplying contraception before sexual intercourse. But still the aim is the same, as is the mechanism and the result.

Very early methods of abortion include 'menstrual regulation' whereby the uterus is emptied shortly after a missed period. Once again the *Offences Against the Person Act* makes this illegal. A soft plastic tube is inserted into the womb attached to a syringe. When the plunger is withdrawn the negative pressure exerted produces a vacuum, which in turn sucks out the contents of the uterus. Until the fragments of tissue are examined afterwards there is no way of knowing whether the woman was pregnant or not; some would rather not know. Some women's groups have learned to do this on themselves and call in the 'gentle method'. New medical (as opposed to surgical) abortifacient agents would include the pill from France, RU240.

First-Trimester Abortion
The vast majority of abortion operations in hospital or clinic are performed at a later stage than the above. They are broadly divided into first and second (or mid) trimester terminations, the cut-off between these two groups lying somewhere between 12 and 14 weeks gestation. The term

'fetus' will from here on be used to refer to the unborn child. Prior to 8 weeks it is an embryo, that is, essential organs such as heart or brain are still being formed, subsequently the change is simply one of growth; and this at an incredible rate. For instance, the length of the fetus doubles from 4 inches to over 8 inches between 12 and 20 weeks. In the first-trimester abortion is safe for the woman via the vaginal route. Over 80 per cent of abortions performed in the UK are first-trimester and most of these are for 'social' reasons.

Patients may be referred to hospital via the general practitioner, or self-referred to a private clinic. The choice of facility depends upon what is available locally, the personal leanings of NHS doctors, and the desire for secrecy. Hospital admission, if only for the day, is necessary, as most operations are performed under general anaesthesia. Abortion cases frequently figure on an ordinary gynaecological list, along with hysterectomies, 'repairs' and D & Cs. The same ward may contain patients undergoing investigation for infertility and abortion cases in adjacent beds (though a humane Sister will try to avoid this).

The operation of vacuum aspiration is, in itself, usually straightforward and over and done with in a matter of 5 or 10 minutes. The cervix, the neck of the womb, is dilated (as for D & C) by passing metal instruments of graduated diameter through its opening. The degree of dilatation required will depend on the size of pregnancy to be aborted. During this procedure the bag of waters is broken; the fetus and placenta (afterbirth) are then removed by suction. The 'sucker' is a hollow instrument made of metal or plastic which fits on to a length of plastic tubing and is then passed into the womb. The other end of the plastic tubing is attached to a large glass bottle within which a vacuum is created via another attachment; thus the contents of the uterus end up in the bottle. The amount of blood lost during this operation can be surprisingly great, amounting to a pint or more.

Immediate risks other than haemorrhage include perforation of the uterus (which in extreme case could lead to hysterectomy), the introduction of infection with the possibility of later infertility due to blocked tubes, and 'retained products' - that is retention of fragments of placenta, causing further bleeding and susceptibility to infection. In spite of these, we are reassured that current figures show early abortion in experienced (or at least supervised) hands, in the short and long-term to be safe. '. . . a mortality rate of less than 1/100,000 operations . . . similar to the risk of dying from an injection of penicillin' quotes a well-known (pro-abortion) gynaecologist.[2]

Second-Trimester Abortion

In the private sector, abortion even beyond 20 weeks is performed in a manner similar to that described above. Naturally the cervix requires dilatation to a larger size, and the fetus, because it is so much bigger, has to be removed piecemeal: it could not possibly pass down the suction tube. The portion of the baby causing most difficulty for the operator is the head. The bones are much harder by this stage and a fragment of skull may easily perforate the uterine wall with serious consequences.

Mid-trimester abortion in NHS hospitals generally involves the use of prostaglandin drugs. Prostaglandins are naturally occurring, hormone-like substances which are produced in various parts of the body; they are short-lived and act at the site of their production. Different ones are being isolated all the time, and they can now be synthesised. Prostaglandins are available for administration in four principal forms for obstetric and gynaecological use: intravenous drip, intra-amniotic injection, and extra-amniotic drip. Vaginal pessaries are sometimes used in early abortion cases to soften the cervix, making it easier to dilate, particularly when it is a first pregnancy in a young girl. In late termination however, the choice usually lies between the intra- and extra-amniotic routes.

2. Wendy Savage, 'Abortion: methods and sequelae', *British Journal of Hospital Medicine*, October, 1982, p. 364.

The intra-amniotic injection is made directly into the womb through the front of the abdomen. Some of the baby's water is removed, and the drug then injected. This method works quickly, the patient experiences labour and delivers the fetus, often within 6 hours. The extra-amniotic method, on the other hand, takes longer. The drug is passed up through a tube in the cervix where it is deposited in the space between the bag of waters and the uterine wall. These patients may labour for up to 48 hours or even longer. Abortion at this gestation often results in the retention of a greater or lesser amount of the afterbirth and a D & C type of procedure is routinely performed to remove this.

Prostaglandins as such do not necessarily kill the fetus; its immaturity, even at 20 to 22 weeks usually results in death during labour or delivery (as in spontaneously occurring miscarriages at this relatively late stage). The further advanced the pregnancy, though, the more likely is a live birth: that is, a heart beat, with or without breathing efforts, is present in the baby at delivery. This is an embarrassment to the abortionist and techniques have been devised to ensure that it does not happen. Concentrated salt solution (saline) or urea injected directly into the womb are occasionally used to kill the baby when there is a greater 'risk' that it may be born alive.

Most gynaecologists have their own arbitrary cut-off point beyond which they will not perform abortions. The illogicality of this has been implied already - what is the difference between a 12 weeks and 24, other than size? These days an ultrasound scan should resolve any doubts there may be concerning the dates, for gestational assessment is accurate to within a few days. This makes causes such as the 'Luton baby' all the more unbelievable; a child of over 30 weeks gestation was delivered as a 'prostaglandin abortion' and, not surprisingly, lived.

Prior to the prostaglandin era hysterotomy was frequently used. It is an operation similar to caesarean section though the uterus is opened in its upper portion rather than the lower. The scar of the hysterotomy incision has the propensity to give way, making subsequent pregnancies more hazardous. Hysterotomy was frequently combined with sterilisation. The impression that many of the late abortions are performed because of fetal abnormality proves false when the overall statistics are examined. It is seen that these account for only about a tenth; the rest are for social indications.

Antenatal Screening
'Screening' implies testing a given population for a particular disease, for example pre-cancerous conditions of the cervix. In the pregnant woman blood tests are done to screen for anaemia, abnormal antibodies and so on. The unborn child is also screened for abnormalities but in this case so often the aim is to kill rather than cure.

The most widely used tests are for spina bifida and mongolism (Down's syndrome). Spina bifida (or neural tube defect) develops in embryonic life as a failure in formation of the spine. A hollow structure, the neural tube, remains open exposing the delicate nerve tissue normally supplying the lower part of the body. This condition varies enormously in severity, the milder cases leading a completely normal life, the most severe dying at birth. Those of moderate severity may be helped by surgery. Spina bifida has a geographical distribution, becoming commoner further north in this hemisphere, and within Britain there are certain black spots such as South Wales.

The precise cause is still unknown but recent research has shown that there is a nutritional element. Pregnant women receiving vitamin supplements before and during early pregnancy show a significantly reduced incidence of the condition. This is all well and good for planned pregnancies, but what about the rest? Screening tests are applied to all women in some hospitals, but only to those at risk (such as a family history of defect) in others. The traditional tests for spina bifida depend on the detection of a substance called alpha-feto-protein (AFP) found in amniotic fluid and the mother's blood. Interpretation of the results depends on ac-

77

curate gestational dating, so in addition the woman must have an ultrasound scan to verify her last menstrual period date.

The blood test is performed at around 12 to 14 weeks; an abnormal result would normally indicate the need for amniocentesis. Where at-risk women alone are investigated they usually proceed directly to amniocentesis at 16 weeks. The method of removing the fluid from the womb is very similar to that used for intra-amniotic prostaglandin abortion. A needle is pushed through the lower part of the abdomen straight into the uterus, generally under strict ultrasound control to avoid damage to the baby or afterbirth; even so the risk of miscarriage lies somewhere between a half and one percent. It goes without saying that the woman must understand that should the result of her test prove abnormal she will undergo abortion. There is little point in carrying out any investigation if its result makes no difference to the management of the case.

When considering the test for Down's syndrome the implication of abortion is even more important, for the investigation is a lengthy, costly affair. The baby's cells, after removal in the amniotic fluid sample, are cultured, then microscopically examined during cell division. The cell nucleus contains the chromosomes, tiny strands carrying the genetic material. These are examined by highly trained experts in the field of genetics and a result is usually available within three weeks or so. Down's syndrome is caused by the presence of one extra chromosome, over and above the normal number of 46. Similar syndromes are the result of portions of a choromosome being missing or misplaced. Older women expecting a baby are offered this test as the incidence of mongolism rises in the late 30s and more markedly in the 40s.

It is interesting that the incidence of babies born each year with Down's syndrome has remained largely unchanged in spite of screening. This is because the vast majority of babies are born to younger women in whom there is also a natural incidence of this defect. With spina bifida the story is very different. There has been a steady decline in the number of babies born with this complaint. This reduction in numbers has been greater than would be expected even taking into consideration the number of neural tube defect cases aborted, and allowing for those who may have received the vitamin therapy. It seems that the actual incidence of spina bifida is decreasing for reasons that cannot be explained.

Amniocentesis as a diagnostic tool for spina bifida may be on the wane. Ultrasound techniques are improving all the time and scanning alone will probably soon replace the present invasive methods of investigation. It is now possible to examine the unborn child minutely and, on a positive note, scanning is applied for many purposes other than the destruction of the abnormal child. Defects in the baby which are amenable to surgery can be diagnosed and treated.

A further development has been fetoscopy. The fetoscope is a fine telescope which is inserted directly into the uterus, allowing visualization of the fetus. Abnormalities of limbs, face, spine are seen and those babies not measuring up to 'normal' are aborted. Fetoscopy is not generally available, nor is it likely to be, as its use demands an extra level of specialist training on the part of the operator. The technique has been developed chiefly to enable safer, more accurate sampling of the baby's blood to diagnose a condition called thalassaemia. This blood disorder afflicts certain Mediterranean populations; it is not lethal at birth, but severely affected children usually die during childhood. The ultimate aim of fetoscopy is to kill the child before it gets even that far. The advance in treatment for thalassaemia has surely been held back by such an attitude.

Finally, some less commonly used, but in other ways more sinister, applications of antenatal diagnosis include 'wrong sex' abortion. Amniocentesis and chromosome analysis, as an incidental, provide the sex of the baby before birth. This has been used in the management of patients in whom there is a high risk of producing a child with a 'sex linked' disorder, such as muscular dystrophy. The fetus, if male, is aborted. However, a *normal* child, simply because it is not of the sex desired by the parents is sometimes aborted.

In the same manner that AFP screening is being super-seded by better ultrasound, so it appears that amniocentesis for Down's may be replaced in the not too distant future. Chorion villus biopsy is a technique of obtaining early pla-cental tissue during the first 2 months or so of pregnancy. Fetal cells are then cultured for genetic study, as described above. The 'advantages' are that the woman is saved a mid-trimester abortion and may get on with trying again, if she wishes.

Complications and After-Effects of Abortion (Sequelae)

Pro-life supporters have, in former years, been able to make much of this factor. But we need to be careful. Abortions done in the early 1970s cannot be properly compared with those performed a decade later. Techniques have been 'improving' all the time, in an attempt to reduce the risks to the mother, both immediate and long-term. It is very difficult to make sense of the medical literature; it abounds with re-ports from all over the world, many drawing conclusions which tally more with the author's moral view on the matter of abortion than with scientific evidence. There are few 'prospective' studies, most are 'retrospective', that is they look back at hospital records, or send out questionnaires to women who have already had an abortion. To prove that abortion has the detrimental effects we suppose, a group undergoing abortion has to be exactly matched for age, social class, marital status, number of previous pregnancies, sexual habits, contraceptive usage, smoking habits, etc., with an-other group not having an abortion. Then one has to decide whether to compare the abortion group with women who have had a spontaneous miscarriage or no pregnancy at all. These groups of women may now be followed into the fu-ture.[3]

3. Such a Study has recently published its first report; it was the com-bined work of the Royal Colleges of Obstetricians and Gynaecolo-

Immediate complications

These can be broadly divided into bleeding and infection. The pregnant uterus is an extremely vascular structure, there is a dramatic increase in the amount of blood circulating through it. From early on the pulse rate of the pregnant woman has increased and the heart is actually putting out more blood with each beat: all to accommodate the tiny fetus which is growing at a phenomenal rate. The wall of the womb is much softer than in the non-pregnant state; a termination, even an early one, is not strictly comparable with a D & C, though the same sort of instruments are used. Bleeding at operation arises from where the afterbirth was situated, but it may be excessive if the wall of the uterus is damaged. An abdominal operation to repair the defect or even hysterectomy may become necessary. Bleeding sometimes arises from the cervix. It can be particularly difficult to dilate in a young girl. The very cases where the argument for abortion may seem the strongest are those in whom damage to the cervix is the most likely.

Infection is probably most commonly associated with fragments of placenta left behind in the womb. A quiescent infection is sometimes present in the fallopian tubes before operation, and this is activated by the abortion, resulting in salpingitis (infection in the tubes) afterwards. These cases are particularly at risk of becoming infertile. Modern antibiotics prevent the deaths of years ago but often cannot eradicate completely the milder sort of pelvic infection which leads to menstrual irregularities and chronic pain in later life.

gists, and General Practitioners (RCOG/RCGP), *Journal of the Royal College of General Practitioners*, April 1985, pp. 175-180.

Long-term complications

These are the cause of more controversy in the literature than the immediate ones. They subdivide principally into problems of fertility and difficulties in carrying a future pregnancy. Infection has already been discussed and is a potent cause of tubal blockage. Some reports also show a higher incidence of ectopic pregnancy after abortion. Note, however, that these problems are more prevalent in any case in a population which is sexually permissive; both 'ordinary' and venereal infections can be contracted without having had an abortion. Spontaneous abortion, and premature birth are all said to be commoner in women who have had a previous termination, though again it may reflect the patient's socio-economic background as much as anything else. The comprehensive review by Wendy Savage[4] suggests that a first-trimester abortion, performed by the vacuum aspiration method, does not increase the risk of a future first-trimester miscarriage, though it is conceded that mid-trimester losses may be as much as doubled. The combined RCOG/RCGP study[5] shows no statistical long-term physical risk in early abortion.

One of the most difficult aspects to follow up is the psychological. Deep, long-lasting depression may frequently result from abortion, and this may not be known to the doctors who performed the operation. The woman herself may not acknowledge it for years. Anecdotal instances abound where guilt feelings surface at Christian conversion. The deep down 'gut reaction' of most women is that abortion is wrong, yet they are persuaded by this present generation (often the professionals) that it is right.

4. Wendy Savage, *op. cit.*
5. RCOG/RCGP Study, as above.

Problem Areas

Mother's life

What if there is a stark choice between the mother's life and the baby's? In reality, thanks to modern medicine, this is a situation which almost never arises. Those genuine cases of severe blood pressure, kidney disease or unstable diabetes can, with the appropriate medical specialist care, often be brought to viability. The term 'viability' denotes the gestational age at which babies generally survive outside the womb. As each year passes this age falls, 26-week-old ones regularly live these days and, more exceptionally, younger still. A pregnancy may quite properly be terminated for maternal reasons, but the aim is to save *both* patients. Note that when an abortion is performed it is with the express intention of killing the unborn child.

A paper published by Murphy and O'Driscoll[6] sets out to examine the maternal deaths over a 10-year period, to determine how many deaths could be directly attributed to the pregnancy: this in a land where abortion is illegal. Amongst 70,000 births there were only three deaths which were due to chronic disease in the mother, though it is doubtful whether two of them would have been saved by early abortion as they were due to conditions not apparent in early pregnancy. They were therefore left with *one* case. This woman had a serious heart defect and was advised against having a baby. She nevertheless embarked upon pregnancy and, sadly, died after the delivery of her baby who survived. This case exemplifies the situation not infrequently encountered where those very women in whom one could justifiably consider abortion on strictly medical grounds, are the ones who will refuse it in any case.

Where the stark choice remains, however, the Christian response must surely be to save the mother. If the preg-

6. J. F. Murphy and K. O'Driscoll, 'Therapeutic Abortion: The Medical Argument', *Irish Medical Journal*, August 1982, vol. 75, pp. 304 ff.

nancy is not far advanced her death will automatically result in the loss of the baby too. There are occasions, for example, cancer of the cervix diagnosed early in the pregnancy, where the normal treatment should be given. This will *incidentally* kill the fetus, whether it is hysterectomy or radiotherapy.

Rape and incest

This problem is more academic than actual as pregnancy resultant upon such assaults is rather unusual, but no-one can pretend that there is an easy answer to this difficult situation. It is argued that here the post-coital forms of 'contraception' lend themselves ideally, provided the victim presents herself soon enough. Abortion as such will not undo the evil already done and in a sense it is only another assault upon the woman, adding to the psychological and physical harm already suffered. There are anecdotal cases where a child conceived by rape or incest has been a blessing.

Anencephaly

This fetal condition stands on its own. It is always incompatible with life outside the womb, though the child may survive some hours after birth. The anencephalic fetus develops without a proper head; there is a face but little else, and the condition is frequently associated with spina bifida. Routine ultrasound scanning in early pregnancy will usually define the condition. The question then is - does the doctor sit back and watch his patient for the next 5 months until she delivers naturally, or does he intervene? How would the woman feel knowing all those weeks that the child she is carrying is doomed? It would seem that the Christian response should allow for termination of such a pregnancy. Yet a case is known to the author of a patient having such guilt feelings from an earlier abortion that she knowingly carried an anencephalic to term.

The 'population explosion'

This provides an argument in favour of methods of 'contraception' such as the IUD, with abortion to fall back on. The widely held supposition that the population would 'explode' without these measures has been widely challenged. Fluctuations in population took place in Europe well before 'family planning' arrived on the scene, with an overall downward trend.

Eastern bloc countries have had the most liberal abortion laws for the longest time. In a country such as Rumania it would not be uncommon to find women who have had 20 or so abortions. But what has happened? Populations are dwindling, and around the world abortion laws are being repealed. The EEC is currently facing the problem and various member countries, such as France, are inducing couples to have more children by financial incentives.

Return to the 'back-street'

The spectre of a step back into recent history, the era of septic abortions due to implements such as coathangers, has put many thinking people off the idea of repealing our laws to make abortion illegal again. The truth of the matter is that this would be most unlikely. There would probably soon be (and maybe already is) a thriving back-street trade in modern abortifacient agents. This in addition to the simpler suction methods. Medical abortion may soon be available through the high street chemists in any case, as the 'do-it-yourself' kits arrive on the market.

Whether we start with scientific and medical facts and examine them in the light of scripture, or indeed begin with a study of the biblical principles and apply them to our present day knowledge and abortion practices, we find that there is a big discrepancy between God's standards and what is actually happening. On the one hand science endorses the Christian view, held through the ages until recent decades, that human life starts at conception, yet on the other it is devising yet more efficient ways of terminating pregnancy.

Many Christians think that abortion does not involve them, yet most of us have someone within our own circle of family or friends whose life has been touched by this event. If we take the trouble to make a study of the subject and see what God has to say about it, we will usually be convinced of the evil of abortion. Having reached this position we then need to back up our words with practical action. There are several pro-life agencies to choose from and it is our duty, as Christians, to be involved.

LIFE ISSUES (2): INFANTICIDE

Ian L. Brown

Introduction

Infanticide is defined in the *Concise Oxford Dictionary* as the killing of an infant soon after birth especially with the mother's consent. This is the sense in which the term is used in English Law, but the more general usage is of the killing of a child after birth by any person or persons. In this chapter the term is used synonymously with 'euthanasia' but with special application to the death of infants.

Until 1981 the general public in the United Kingdom had little knowledge that infanticide could be occurring in this country. However, in the early summer of 1981 two cases came to public attention in which the lives of infants with Down's syndrome (mongolism) received diametrically opposed treatment and resulted in the doctor involved in one of the cases being charged with murder. Using these two cases as an introduction to illustrate the complexities of current clinical practice in paediatric hospitals I shall outline the problems inherent in the management of 'defective' children from the point of view of the medical profession, the parents and society.

Further background to the publicity which these cases received may be seen in a brief consideration of the 1980 Reith Lectures given by Ian Kennedy and entitled 'Unmasking Medicine'. In these lectures the whole problem of the moral and social accountability of the medical profession was discussed, Kennedy's thesis being that for too long the public has accepted the doctor's right to (almost) absolute power and secrecy in the clinical situation and as a result medicine has become autocratic, authoritarian and self-serving. The National Health Service is a 'National Illness Service' and those who are most affected by doctors' decisions - the patients - have no right to discuss or demand an explanation regarding treatment or non-treatment. The medical profession makes ethical decisions regarding clinical situations with little, if any, consideration of wider public opinion. Whatever the validity of these opinions, the Lectures resulted in a greater awareness in medical circles of outside interest and concern with ethical problems long thought to be purely of concern to the medical profession. Since then there has been much wider interest in the 'performance' of doctors and this has been reflected in increased litigation against medical practitioners by patients or their relatives to receive redress for errors in medical practice. The concept of confidentiality has been widely discussed, and computerisation of medical records has been complicated by the introduction of the Data Protection Act.

The Problem of Infanticide

The two cases
The first case is that of a baby girl born with Down's syndrome (mongolism), complicated by intestinal obstruction. Down's syndrome is a congenital abnormality caused by an alteration in the structure of the genetic material (usually affecting chromosome 21), which results in various relatively minor physical defects (such as the characteristic 'mongoloid' face, enlarged tongue, abnormal skin creases on the palm of the hand) and degrees of mental impairment. Such children are usually physically healthy at birth and the condition may not be recognised immediately (as distinct from spina bifida, which is easily recognised at birth). In addition mongol children have a higher incidence of other physical defects at birth, such as intestinal atresia (failure of correct development of the intestine which will result in bowel obstruction), which also occur almost at random in the population. Operations to relieve intestinal obstructions due to atresia are performed routinely on neonates with very good results.

A decision therefore *not* to treat a baby with a surgically correctable obstruction solely on the grounds that she is a mongol is to imply that she may be better off dead simply because she is mongol. The dilemma is, of course, that until fairly recently, a baby with intestinal obstruction would have died, and it is the availability of sophisticated anaesthesia, paediatric intensive care units and reliable surgical techniques which have created the problem. The existence of a particular treatment does not, of course, mean that it *must* or even should be used in all circumstances, but this then implies a value judgment to assess who should receive treatment.

The additional complication in this case was that the parents had decided that they did not want the child: 'Alexandra's parents said that nature had "made its own arrangements to terminate a life which could not be fruitful".'[1]

The case was taken to the Court of Appeal which decided that society had a responsibility to the infant, and a successful operation was performed. A leading article in the *British Medical Journal* had this to say about the case: 'But do we want a society where "fruitfulness", in however wide a sense, determines worth or the right to live?. . . The ultimate decisions about life or death are not simply medical decisions.'[2]

The second case concerned the trial of Dr Leonard Arthur at Leicester Crown Court for the murder of John Pearson, born with Down's syndrome on 28 June, 1980. The baby died 69 hours later with a level of the drug dihydrocodeine (used as a sedative) more than twice the lethal adult dose in his body. The story in this case makes somewhat sordid reading. An anonymous informer at Derby City Hospital reported the death to Life and thence to the police alleging the child's death was caused by the doctor. The charge of murder was changed to attempted murder when the prosecution's leading expert witness was forced by defence evidence to withdraw his statement that the baby had a normal brain - there was evidence of birth injury to the brain. This change of emphasis moved the chief focus of attention from the *cause* of the baby's death to Dr Arthur's *intention* in his clinical management of the case. The judge directed the

1. *British Medical Journal*, 1981, 283, pp. 569-570.
2. *Ibid.*

jury that what mattered was not Dr Arthur's motives, but whether the intention of the treatment was to cause John Pearson's death. The decision was not guilty of attempted murder.

Much has been made of this case as setting a legal precedent which will allow doctors to act with impunity under the law. The *Sunday Times* on 8 November, 1981, stated that the jury's verdict enclosed the 'principle' that it is kinder to allow a severely handicapped and unwanted baby to die than to help it to live. The medico-legal correspondent of the *British Medical Journal* had this to say on the decision: 'The case of R. *v*. Arthur has decided one matter only: that Dr Arthur was not guilty of murder or attempted murder. It is wrong to argue that any kind of legal history has been made by the decision . . . .'

During the detailed reporting of this case in the press current practice in dealing with handicapped infants was fully exposed to public attention. In the next section we will examine some of the methods of treatment in use and discuss their effects.

Medical care of the defective infant

When a baby is born with a physical defect, be it a condition such as Down's syndrome, or a heart malformation, or failure of the abdominal wall to close in the uterus allowing the intestines to remain outside the abdomen, or where spina bifida is present, three considerations are immediately apparent:

1. The parents must be counselled regarding the future of their child;
2. Clinical decisions must be taken regarding the clinical management of the child;
3. The potential burden on society must be assessed.

It is, however, just at this point that all three of these considerations are most difficult to assess. The parents obviously will be emotionally drained, and often suffer a bereavement-like reaction, including rejection of the facts and guilt feelings. The doctors involved are faced with decisions which may involve lengthy operations and difficult nursing management problems, often with inadequate resources at their disposal. And who can assess what society is willing to bear in terms of emotional and financial commitment to the handicapped?

There are three clinical options open to the doctor in such cases as those described above:

1. Full surgical and medical intervention is undertaken to correct remediable defects, and every effort is made to maintain the infant's life.
2. No surgical intervention is undertaken and the baby receives nursing care only.
3. The baby is not treated or cared for and is allowed to die, 'nature' taking its course.

A fourth option would, of course, be actually to take the infant's life by active intervention with drugs - this would legally be regarded as murder, and is not generally considered as a suitable or acceptable clinical option.

Until fairly recently, option 1 above would have been the only one most paediatricians would consider. However, the other two options are currently regarded as suitable and acceptable in clinical practice, and option 2 is widely used in neonatal clinics. It will be considered in detail at this stage.

The concept of 'nursing care only'
Following the trial of Dr Arthur the concept of 'nursing care only' was discussed in depth in the correspondence columns of *The Lancet* and the *British Medical Journal* and in their editorials. In this section quotations are presented from these journals and their implications discussed, in order to present what is seen as 'standard' medical practice in this field. The discussion will be broadened to deal with practice in the USA later.

The Lancet's editorial of November 14, 1981 had this to say:

> Respected physicians declared at the trial that 'nursing care only' is within the spectrum of acceptable management for Down's syndrome without additional handicap. Such a course can lead to slow and distressful death, but is nevertheless pursued because rapidly lethal 'treatment' is believed to be unethical as well as illegal . . . . But do the advocates of 'nursing care only' advise parents on the quality of death?[3]

This concept of the 'quality of death' has been dealt with in another chapter of this book in relation to the topic of euthanasia as it applies to adults. It is, of course, easier to consider the quality of human experience as it relates to adult experience and expectations - we all know how *we* would like to be treated as persons, but it is difficult to apply that knowledge to the experience of a twelve hour neonate.

The decision to pursue 'nursing care only' as the line of management of a defective infant is usually taken very soon after birth, and the instructions are given to the nurses involved to proceed with such treatment. What is involved in 'nursing care only'? Herein lies the major difficulty - does nursing care involve only cleaning the baby, adjusting its position in its cot to ensure its comfort, or does it involve feeding? Professor Zachary, a leading British paediatrician, writes:

> The order 'nursing care only' was interpreted by the nursing staff (and they were not corrected in this interpretation) as meaning that no milk feeds should be offered; yet perhaps half the work of the nurse on a neonatal ward is taken up with feeding infants.[4]

If the baby is not fed, does this imply enforced starvation? Indeed, withholding food may be regarded as an active course to hasten death. The withholding of nutrition is not

3. *The Lancet*, 1981, ii, pp. 1085-1086.
4. *British Medical Journal*, 1981, 283, p. 1463.

accepted in other branches of medicine as ethical treatment - and even patients with terminal cancer are fed, great effort being expended to supply a suitable, palatable diet for the dying patient. What is the difference between a defective neonate and an adult with terminal disease? An article in *The Lancet*[5] suggested that the newborn baby did not actually qualify as a human being, but only as a 'potential' person. We are used in post-Warnock days to hearing the embryo described in these terms, but not a baby: this article was published in 1979, and reflects how far medical ethics had slipped even then. If a normal neonate does not qualify as a member of the human race, what hope is there for a defective child? Editorial comment in *The Lancet*[6] referred to this earlier article: 'This argument, of course, is a slippery slope which might end in the despatch of babies with red hair, or girls.'

There was another aspect of the Arthur case which caused disquiet: the Home Office pathologist, Professor Alan Usher, found that the baby died due to poisoning with the drug dihydrocodeine given in a dose of 5mg as a sedative (this dose is larger than that recommended for a child of over 4 years) which resulted in a level of the drug slightly more than twice the average fatal level for adults in the baby's blood.

Is there a single paediatrician in the country who would administer dihydrocodeine in doses of 5mg as a sedative to his own newborn baby? The sight of several distinguished physicians (including the President of the Royal College of Physicians) agreeing with the administration of this dose of drug for 'suffering and pain', when they must know that the neonate with apparently uncomplicated Down's syndrome has no suffering or pain whatever must make one doubt whether they would agree with your dictum about dying 'by default' let alone by the positive action of a drug which must be lethal and for which there is no clinical indication.[7]

5. *The Lancet*, 1979, ii, pp. 1123-1124.
6. *The Lancet*, 1981, ii, pp. 1085-1086.
7. *British Medical Journal*, 1981, 283.

The concept of 'nursing care only' therefore appears to imply total rejection of the infant which is not fed and the administration of potentially lethal drugs with no clinical indication, and in doses ten times those recommended in standard texts. In other words the option of 'nursing care only' means allowing the child to die, with a 'built-in insurance policy guaranteeing the correctness of the forecast by giving the babies heavy doses of hypnotic drugs'.[8]

There seems little difference between option 2 above, *i.e.* 'nursing care only', and option 3, allowing the baby to die. Indeed the administration of sedative drugs in the doses reported suggests the ethically and legally unacceptable alternative step of actively intervening to procure the infant's death. There have been several legal cases in recent years in which doctors have been sued for the *accidental* administration of excessive doses of drugs including antibiotics which have resulted in deafness or some other severe side effect. Large amounts of financial compensation have been awarded to parents and victims for these accidents, yet no-one has attempted to sue on the basis of the administration of unjustifiable levels of drugs causing the death of a defective baby. Why is this? Surely it is because we regard the abnormal infant as being sub-human, unable to develop its full human potential, a life of 'fruitfulness'. How do we define human fruitfulness?

At this stage we could with some justification redefine 'infanticide' as 'infant euthanasia', for that is what we are describing:

> Preservation at all costs is the one way to satisfy those who believe that the acquittal of Dr Arthur has opened the path to the widespread acceptance of euthanasia as an estimable feature of modern society. For those who condemn euthanasia or non-treatment, the issue is simple: no doctor must ever do less than his utmost to preserve life.[9]

8. Quoted in *Biblical/Medical Ethics*, F. E. Payne, Michigan, 1985.
9. *The Lancet, op. cit.*

So far we have dealt only with the situation as it appears in the UK. Do other countries have a similar attitude to neonatal problems? In the USA the case equivalent to the ones we have discussed is referred to as the 'Baby Doe' case. Baby Doe was born on 9 April 1982 with Down's syndrome and oesophageal atresia correctable by surgery. She died on 15 April of starvation, because her parents and doctors decided to withhold surgical treatment. Their decision was upheld by the Indiana Supreme Court, the parents' lawyer having said: 'We are not dealing with a condemnation of death, we are dealing with two appropriate methods of treatment for a very sad case.'[10]

Baby Doe was not unique in American experience except that, as in the two British cases described above, legal decisions were required to 'sanctify' what were already established procedures in the hospitals concerned. One report indicates that forty-three babies were allowed to die following discussion between doctors and parents in a 30 month period.[11]

The approach to the issue of the defective child seems to be identical on both sides of the Atlantic. In the next section of this chapter we will explore the ethical issues with regard to infanticide and seek a biblical approach to them.

The Right to Live and the Right to Die
This is the title of the *British Medical Journal* editorial of 29 August 1981,[12] which contains the statement: 'The ultimate decisions about life and death are not simply medical decisions.'

Why have we seen in the last few years these dramatic changes in medical practice which the development of 'infant euthanasia' represents? The *British Medical Journal* appears

10. Payne, *op. cit.*
11. R. S. Duff, A. G. Campbell, 'Moral and Ethical Dilemmas in the Special Care Nursery', *New England Journal of Medicine*, 1983, 289, pp. 890-894.
12. *British Medical Journal*, 1981, 283, pp. 569-570.

to have the answer to this question: 'We believe that in the absence of a clear code to which society adheres . . . .'[13]

The concept of a societal ethical code and of quality of life have been dealt with in other chapters, but they are perhaps most obviously relevant in our discussion of the treatment of defective infants. Quality of life is the point at issue in this debate.

Quality of life is very difficult to define, and depends to a great extent on what society anticipates that a satisfying, fruitful life will include. It is not therefore translatable between different societies. I may anticipate continued employment, a satisfying professional life, a high salary, two cars, private education for my children and a comfortable retirement in a country cottage, as being an adequate quality of life. For many others in this country quality of life would be enhanced by any employment, diminished debt and adequate heating in the winter. In other countries quality of life might be improved by equal opportunities for all races, or the right to vote, or enough food to live above starvation level, to avoid the pot-belly of kwashiorkor. My anticipated quality of life is totally irrelevant to the Sudanese refugee, or the child of Soweto.

Quality of life may also vary at different times in one's life: when I was a student I ate pie and beans each day in the hospital canteen; now I am a doctor and I concentrate on chicken curry and roast beef and Yorkshire pudding! These are facetious illustrations, but they make the point that quality of life is entirely arbitrary and subjective. It depends on private experience and desires and is essentially a selfish concept, since my quality of life can usually only be sustained at the expense of another's. There is no objective way of assessing quality of life, nor of establishing criteria for it which would be universally acceptable.

In effect, when I assess the potential fruitfulness of a baby with Down's syndrome or spina bifida, I decide that as a normal fit adult male with a satisfying and stimulating ca-

13. *Ibid.*

reer the baby will not be able to enjoy *my* quality of life and hence that baby will not enjoy its own potential life and experience. Its life will not be meaningful in *my* eyes and therefore it has no right (or need) to life.

We are placed in the situation of making value-judgments regarding quality of life based not on any set, external standard or yard-stick but based entirely on personal experience and expectation, *i.e.* on a 'standard' which is entirely fluid and which has no fixed point of reference. Also, having decided that the quality of life will be so low as not to justify existing at all, we cannot ask the person concerned (the neonate) whether they approve of the decision or not. Perhaps he or she would have chosen limited life rather than death. Who can tell?

In fact the concept of quality of life applies more to the parents' expectations for *their* lives than to the infant's life in many cases. It is the effect that the responsibility for a defective child will have on the parents and other family members that is often given prime consideration. Indeed the reactions and capabilities of the parents must be considered and the strength of the family assessed before expecting them to accept wholeheartedly the misfortune which has befallen them. Yet many families with abnormal children testify to the joy they have experienced in coping with and caring for their handicapped child, and significant numbers of children with Down's syndrome survive into adult life and may even become established authors.[14]

On the other hand, if we are to suggest that full and effective treatment be given to infants with remedial defects, then we must as a society be willing to pay the cost in terms of commitment to their maintenance which may involve long-term nursing, institutional care, *etc*. If parents are willing to care for the child, adequate help must be available from society to allow for holidays, to help with housing alterations, baby-sitting, transport. If the natural parents are unwilling to

14. *British Medical Journal*, 1981, 283, p. 1463.

keep the child, then fostering or adoption are still viable alternatives which must be pursued.

What are the parents' rights in these situations? Having conceived the child, do the parents have rights as well as responsibilities? The British Medical Association has made the following comment:

> All patients have identical rights whether they are in their teens, aged 70, or infants - one right is to accept or reject medical treatment. For example, doctors may offer an elderly patient an operation for cancer. The patient may decide to refuse surgery and ask to be cared for at home with the family, letting the disease take its natural course with appropriate medication from the GP. Similarly, a newborn baby has the right to accept or reject treatment. As the infant cannot take the decision personally it is the responsibility of the parents to take the decision. The decision will be based on consultation with the doctors, perhaps the GP, and perhaps a vicar or priest, but the *Handbook of Medical Ethics* quite clearly states, 'The parents must ultimately decide.' It is the doctor's duty to save life, so the balance in difficult cases will be in favour of active medical intervention for the infant. Doctors will agree with the parents' decision to refuse treatment for the infant if they believe that any operation would postpone the inevitable - if surgery would merely put back the baby's death by a short while.[15]

There appears to me to be a certain illogicality in this statement - the infant cannot take the decision, the doctor has a duty to act, the parents must decide, the doctor will agree with the parents. Since the infant cannot say 'yea' or 'nay', surely it must be assumed that he would say 'yea', particularly since the doctor's duty is to act to save life. The majority of major operations, on children or adults, only postpone the inevitable and put death back a variable length of time, yet this argument is not used to defend failure to operate in the majority of cases. Indeed on the basis of this argument one could put forward a case for the abandonment of all therapeutic endeavour, since all must die!

15. *British Medical Journal*, 1981, 283, p. 567.

No, there is something more at stake here. We return again to the issue of the value of the individual human being. The argument has been raised in the context of the abortion issue that the fetus is not human, and we have already quoted the anonymous article in *The Lancet* extending this concept to the neonate.[16]This argument has distinguished antecedents. In 1973 Watson, a Nobel Prize winner, was quoted as saying:

> If a child were not declared alive until three days after birth, then all parents could be allowed the choice only a few are given under the present system. The doctor could allow the child to die if the parents so choose and save a lot of misery and suffering. I believe this view is the only rational, compassionate attitude to have.[17]

Where is the rationality in this statement? If the child be not declared alive, how can it be allowed to die? It must surely just not exist, and it patently does exist and exhibit all the biological features of life. Where is the compassion in this statement? Is it compassionate to allow the child (or whatever it would be called) to die? Who is being saved misery and suffering?

Crick, Watson's Nobel Prize-sharing colleague, added this statement in 1978: 'no newborn infant should be declared human until it has passed certain tests regarding its genetic endowment and that if it fails these tests it forfeits the right to live.'[18]

Who would determine the tests necessary for inclusion in the human race?

There is, therefore, a general feeling among scientists and doctors alike that the presence of a physical or mental defect in an infant in effect excludes that child from the human race. Few would state it so plainly as Watson and Crick

16. *British Medical Journal*, 1981, 283, pp. 569-570.
17. Quoted in *Whatever Happened to the Human Race?*, F. A. Schaeffer, C. E. Koop, London, 1980.
18. *Ibid.*

have done, but that is an acceptable position for rationalist, materialist man to present.

It is our contention that it is the lack of a clear moral and ethical code which allows such statements to be made. Let me now quote more fully from the *British Medical Journal* editorial referred to earlier:

> We believe that in the absence of a clear code to which society adheres there is no justification for usurping parents' rights, or for believing that the courts are more likely to reach a more humane solution. We must beware of that slippery slope that would lead to that nonchalant taking of lives found to be substandard, inconvenient, or expensive; but the 'existence-at-all-costs' view points to a terrain no less treacherous. Letting nature take its course in certain circumstances is to acknowledge that there might sometimes be a right not to live - but we badly need to clear our confusion about what these circumstances are.[19]

All doctors would agree that there are many circumstances where 'masterly inactivity' is to be preferred to aggressive therapeutic intervention; whether there is a right not to live is arguable. As the *BMJ* clearly indicates, if there is no clear societal code on the issue, there is bound to be confusion, indeed chaos, in determining what are allowable circumstances. It is this lack of a clear ethical code which allowed such disparate legal judgments as those described in the two cases at the beginning of this chapter.

The ethical principles which our society adhered to until fairly recently were based on the Judaeo-Christian principles of the intrinsic value of human life - man made in the image of God. A return to this appreciation of the worth of every human being would fill the gap so obviously present in our society. As one letter to the *British Medical Journal* put it:

> With the decline of religion the medical profession has taken over as a moral arbiter. As in the case of your editorial, however, this rarely makes sense. The new teaching that the quality of life as

19. *Ibid.*

judged by other people equals the value of life is the greatest non-sense of all.[20]

It is the Christian's duty to uphold the value of human life over the quality of that life, while struggling to ensure that quality of life is a commodity equally available to all.

20. *British Medical Journal*, 1981, 283, p. 1463.

LIFE ISSUES (3): EUTHANASIA

George L. Chalmers

The term 'euthanasia' derives from two Greek words, *eu* and *thanatos*, which mean, respectively, 'good, easy, right or proper' and 'death'. It therefore means 'good death', or 'dying well' perhaps. If this were the meaning of the term still, there would be little ethical problem, since it is the aim of any doctor who is caring for a dying patient to ensure that they experience as good an end to life as possible, using all the means available to medical skill and science. Good medical care should make the inevitable end of life as easy, gentle and free of distress as it can be.

Unfortunately, the word has come to mean the deliberate termination of someone's life in order to relieve distress and suffering, where the underlying illness cannot be cured. This is, of course, a very different idea, and carries extremely important moral and ethical implications.

The pressure for 'euthanasia'

In the fairly recent past there has been a good deal of pressure for the legalisation of 'euthanasia' in this specific sense of the term. Such pressure has come mainly from a relatively small group calling itself 'Exit', formerly known as the Voluntary Euthanasia Society. These people have gained some measure of publicity, if not support, by the publication of a 'guide to self-release' - a handbook of methods of suicide which might be attempted by someone in the distress of illness which they themselves perceive as terminal.

The principal purpose of the Society remains, however, to maintain pressure for alteration of the law to permit the termination of life in certain circumstances.

They would claim that the law should 'allow, but not compel, doctors to help incurable patients to die peacefully at their own request'. As a safeguard, 'The patient must have signed, at least thirty days previously, a declaration making the request known. The declaration would be independently witnessed by two people, unrelated to the patient, or to each other, who would not stand to gain by the patient's death.' As an additional safeguard the patient would be free to revoke the declaration at any time and medical certification would also be necessary. 'Two doctors, one a consultant, would be required to certify that the person was suffering, without reasonable prospect of recovery, from a physical illness which he found intolerable.'

These extracts from an explanatory leaflet published by Exit might seem at first glance, to be reasonable, but on closer scrutiny and further consideration it is not too difficult to see some problems.

Possible mis-diagnosis or mis-prognosis
Medicine is, on the whole, a scientific profession, but in no sense is it an infallible one. Even with the greatest of care, mis-diagnosis is an ever present possibility, and uncertainties in the area of prognosis are even greater. It is one thing to give a poor prognosis and to be proven wrong by the patient's improvement and survival, but quite another to be proven wrong by the result of a post-mortem examination if the result of your prognosis were a request for euthanasia, subsequently granted and executed.

Difficulties in the definition of terms used
The terms employed in the description of the situation which warrants euthanasia would also produce difficulty. When is a disease 'incurable'? and does that term take into account the possibility of relief without cure? Parkinson's disease might be said to be incurable, but effective treatment will often restore the patient to normal life and function. How does a doctor decide what is a 'reasonable prospect of recovery', especially at a time when new approaches to the relief and management of many diseases are constantly being introduced, often with dramatic effect?

At what point does suffering become 'intolerable', in the light of the major variations in tolerance, not only between people but also in the same person at different times in the context of the same illness?

Problems of objectivity
It is difficult to be objective in making a decision when the outcome *might* be the death of the patient concerned. The difficulties, I suspect would be much more apparent when, by definition, the outcome *will* be the death of another human being - possibly one with whom a very significant personal relationship has been established, in the context of a progressive illness. Death is not an issue in which it is readily possible to become objective, especially in the light of one's own mortality.

Problems of finality
Many medical situations which have gone wrong may be redeemed by the change to a better treatment or management, by the stopping of a toxic medication, or even by the application of patience in observing the course of the illness as it progresses. Once death has occurred, whether 'natural' or induced, there is no way back, no possibility of second thoughts, and no opportunity for a full re-appraisal of the situation.

Difficulties of the 'available option'
Human nature being what it is, and doctors being subject to human nature, there is a very real possibility that what may seem an easy way out will be applied in circumstances which would not be envisaged in the legislation proposed. The option of killing the patient does not exist at present but if it did, might not the doctor be tempted to misuse a provision which would be less demanding than the discipline of good and effective terminal care?

All of these problems arise, even on the briefest consideration of the proposals, and on deeper consideration the issues at stake are readily recognised as fundamental to our concept of the value of human life.

Public support

It is claimed that there is growing support for a change in the law to permit such a procedure, and the claims of compassion are often presented as a warrant for such an opinion. It seems to be little understood that there are better ways of being compassionate than to kill the patient, and it is also important to realise that those who advocate such extreme measures have no monopoly of compassion. It seems unlikely that those responding to random opinion polls, for instance, would have had the time or the opportunity to consider all the implications, and so much depends upon the wording of the questions asked. Many ordinary people will express the wish that suffering should be relieved in terminal illness, and many will also agree that measures to prolong life may be inappropriate where there is little prospect of recovery, but this is a different matter from deciding deliberately to terminate that life.

There is seldom, if ever, any intent on the part of doctors or nurses or anyone else in the caring professions simply to prolong dying or to prolong the suffering of dying. Rather it is the express intention to relieve such distress by all necessary means. It is somewhat ironic that the call for 'euthanasia' legislation comes at a time when resources for the relief of symptoms, including pain, have never been better at any time in history. Compassion may be demonstrated by the careful and informed use of these resources, rather than by the termination of life as a deliberate action. The real aim of terminal care is to have the patient die in comfort when the time comes, rather than to have the patient die at the most convenient time.

'Doctors are doing it anyway'

Those who would support voluntary euthanasia sometimes claim that the termination of life is already carried out by doctors under different guises, and that there is a tacit conspiracy about this which makes the legal situation quite ridiculous.

A small number of doctors have admitted to having agreed to a patient's request that death might be accelerated, and one retired surgeon made some publicity out of this several years ago. In general, however, the members of the healing profession have no desire, whether tacitly or overtly, to become recognised as the killing profession. Such accusation may, however, arise from a misunderstanding of the true facts of the clinical situation.

There are two ways in which the doctor may be misunderstood and be accused of 'doing it anyway'.

He may be seen to discontinue medication which has been previously prescribed for the condition from which the person is suffering, or he may be seen to prescribe medication which is recognisably intended for symptom relief in progressively increasing dosage, even to a level which is stated to be 'lethal' in normal practice.

Discontinued medication, and withheld medication

Medication is given to patients in relation to the specific needs of each patient at a particular point in the course of the illness, and in relation to their pharmacological actions, side-effects and interactions with other treatments. In general, the aim is to promote recovery, and if this aim is being realised a certain measure of discomfort or even hazard may be acceptable, the benefits being held to outweigh the disadvantages. Where a condition is found to be unresponsive to that treatment or even, indeed, to any other treatment, it is not logical or reasonable to continue it, especially if some of its effects are undesirable or unpleasant. Similarly, if it is not to be expected that the medication is likely appreciably to alter the course of the illness, it is better practice not to give it, unless perhaps it is likely to alleviate some of the symptoms. Thus is may be quite sensible to give an antibiotic drug to one terminally ill patient, whose symptoms will be relieved by the control of an infection, and to withhold it from another who has different symptoms from a similar illness. This is a matter of good clinical judgment not, as has been suggested, a form of 'negative euthanasia', with the intent to shorten the patient's life.

In the clinical situation, one seldom, if ever, gives drugs with the specifically defined intention of influencing the patient's life-span, whether to prolong or to reduce it. It is much more usual to prescribe medication to help the patient overcome the illness or, if this is not possible, to relieve the symptoms arising from it. Often the intention is to do both, but one recognises that this is not always possible. The dictum *primum non nocere* - 'first of all we must do no harm' - will often determine whether a particular medicine is given or not.

Inevitably, some tensions must arise in such decisions. These, however, are the tensions for which the doctor's training and experience should be preparing him, and it is very doubtful whether such tensions will be alleviated by changes in the law. Any law which presented the possibility of a less demanding discipline than that of good clinical care for the terminally ill would open the door to a fall in clinical standards, a fall which both profession and public would live (or even die?) to regret.

Analgesia, sedation and 'overdosage'
The use of symptomatic drugs in terminal care is also an area in which there may be misunderstanding. With sedative and analgesic drugs in particular there will sometimes be what is known as a principle of double effect at work.

A particular symptom, *e.g.* pain, may be effectively relieved by a particular group of drugs, *e.g.* the opiates. These drugs have other effects; it is recognised that they may impair the control of breathing, and they may be avoided in most cases where this is a risk. But, if the pain being experienced by the patient is so severe as to cause extreme distress, and if other preparations with less risk have been ineffective, it may be entirely appropriate to prescribe the medication to relieve the pain, accepting the risks in the particular case. Far from being a decision to 'kill the patient with opiates' or even to 'accept that the opiate may kill' this is a decision to relieve the primary clinical problem. This will often result in an improvement, rather than a deterioration in the patient's general condition as well as relieving the pain. This is not to say that opiates are always the best way to do this but it does illustrate the principle. There is a very great difference between active symptomatic treatment and so-called 'disguised euthanasia'. Once again, the exercise of clinical judgment in the light of training and experience is the question at issue.

The matter of dosage of opiates and similar drugs is also raised in the discussion of terminal illness, and instances are quoted of patients who have been seen to receive dosage of such drugs which are sometimes even larger than the recommended upper limits in the text-books. In most instances it will be found on closer enquiry, that these people have been on the preparation for a prolonged time, and have become habituated to the drug. Not only does such a person require higher doses to give relief of symptoms, they also can tolerate these higher doses without additional harm because their bodies have learned to metabolise the drug more efficiently. Thus the toxic effects are less, as well as the symptom relieving effects. The increase in dose is a response to the pharmacological situation, rather than a deliberate attempt to poison the patient.

In general terms it is untrue that 'doctors are doing it anyway'. Most doctors set a high value upon human life and do not wish to be granted the legal 'power of life or death'. Furthermore, even if a small minority could be identified as 'doing it anyway' such action is unquestionably unlawful, identifiably unethical, and a very poor argument for a change in the law which would potentially extend the practice.

Refusal of treatment and the 'living will'

The discussion of euthanasia often raises the matter of the right of a patient to refuse treatment where they do not believe that it will benefit them, or where they do not wish to extend the period of terminal illness. There has also been a good deal of discussion of the so-called 'living will' in which a patient may complete a document forbidding treatment if they should come under medical care in such circumstances as severe dementia, brain damage, or other major disabling illness.

There is, in fact, no obligation upon anyone in law, to accept any form of medical treatment for themselves, and in that sense a refusal of treatment is no more than an exercise of personal freedom. The problem arises when the likely consequences of such a refusal will be the serious deterioration of that person's health and well-being when appropriate treatment might have avoided such deterioration. The desire of the doctor will often be to spare the person the unnecessary trauma of an unrelieved progression of the illness. The doctor may even suspect that the refusal of treatment is the result of a disturbance of thought which may itself be arising from the primary illness. This ought not to be seen as a doctor *v.* patient conflict, in which one party is set to thwart the wishes of the other. In fact, it is often a breakdown in communication, in which emotive issues other than the illness and its management, have been allowed to assume a false priority. These are areas in which a great deal of complex personal interaction is involved. It is well recognised that 'hard cases make bad law' and it seems very probable that a legal involvement in such a situation would offer little apart from further complication.

The 'living will' idea is also based upon very shaky premisses when it is viewed from a clinical point of view. It begs the question of diagnosis in advance and assumes quite falsely a level of prognostic accuracy which it may not be possible to achieve. It also impedes, if applied as it seems to be envisaged, the legitimate application of curative and palliative measures which may be entirely appropriate for the patient concerned at the time of illness.

The effect of legalised euthanasia upon the clinical relationship

The deliberate taking of life, whether by a doctor or by any other person, whether in a situation of terminal illness or otherwise, is an unlawful act, and requires to be recognised as such. The request or consent of the patient, or of anyone else is quite irrelevant.

The doctor, by virtue of his clinical relationship with his patient, is in a position of clear responsibility for the life and health of that patient, and it would be quite inimical to that responsibility for him to be 'licensed to kill'. Such a concept could only undermine and eventually destroy the basic confidence on which the doctor-patient relationship is built.

Some years ago, when a retired surgeon 'confessed' to assisting death in some of his terminal patients, I met a number of old people who were very uncertain about my visit as a hospital specialist lest I was the one who would decide whether they should live or die. I did not enjoy the role in which I was thus unwillingly and unwittingly cast.

'Hanging judges' have been recognised in the past and are remembered with infamy: few practitioners would wish to be defined as 'killing doctors'.

The question of medical motivation

The image of the doctor is sometimes one which suggests total capacity to alter the course of illness at will - to cure the illness by the use of a 'wonder drug' or, indeed, to let it progress by omitting to do so. The 'life or death' situation is seen as his normal milieu and his decision determines the outcome. It is all very black and white, with few shades of grey.

The truth is, in fact very different. Treatment, even well-established treatment, is often, in the individual case, a trial to determine whether a response will follow. Therapy, given with the best intentions, may worsen the situation, while

110

stopping treatment may equally improve it. Medicine remains an art, to a significant extent, notwithstanding the major contribution of science to the management and investigation of disease.

For these reasons, the interpretation of events in terminal illness may boil down to the question, 'What did the doctor intend to achieve?' rather than 'What did the doctor decide should happen?'. Inevitably, the answers become subjective and related to opinion, rather than fact. In the context, if the intent was to hasten death, whether by commission or by omission, this would constitute 'euthanasia' or murder, both in intent and in action. If, on the other hand, the intent were to alleviate symptoms, to avoid complications of treatment, or in some other way to obviate distress, the ethical, and presumably the legal situation would be quite different.

But, again, who can truly determine motive or intent? It is often difficult enough to sort out our own, let alone those of others. It is difficult to escape the subjectivity of the situation, and it is a potential minefield if the law is to become involved in such subjectivity.

Who might be 'candidates' for euthanasia?
The procedure is usually suggested as a possible solution to three kinds of problem:

1. The deformed or impaired child, in whom it is felt that the potential or actual quality of life is so diminished as to make the life no longer worthy of living.

2. The person in middle life with progressive painful or distressing disease, for which there is no specific known cure or treatment and in whom, again, the potential or actual quality of life is diminished.

3. The old person with degenerative disease, neoplastic disease or with severe brain damage or intellectual impairment. In this group there tends to be somewhat

111

more emphasis on the value of the life rather than its quality, and the idea of a 'useless' life is more often entertained.

In each of these groups there are certain assumptions made which may not be entirely valid when applied to the specific instance. How do we decide about whose life is of sufficient quality to be allowed to continue? Who is to make such a decision? Can any individual be entrusted with such a decision about another's life? Can we really envisage a panel or committee which would objectively apply itself to such a question? Could such an individual or even such a committee ever be entirely free of the possibility of error, or of the anxiety about error? By what criteria is the decision to be made? Must we score a certain number of points on an assessment scale, or in some other way meet an objective 'level of unworthiness to live'? Whose consent would be acceptable if the subject's own were unavailable or invalid?

The number of questions raised by the concept itself is legion, and they are matched by the practical difficulties.

If we are to allow the person himself to be the judge, how do we assess the objectivity or the validity of the decision he has made? Many who, in the past, have considered themselves total failures, have proved false in the assessment they have made. Many in the midst of 'incurable' illness have recovered, not only as a result of a new advance in medicine, or of a spontaneous remission in the condition, but also because they have been misinformed about the condition, because they have misinterpreted the facts, or even because the diagnosis has been wrong. If the possibility of error is a strong argument in favour of not killing the guilty, should it not also be heard in respect of the innocent?

The prophet Elijah, in his depressive state, sought the Lord to 'take away' his life, but its quality and value were by no means dissipated at that point.

If, on the other hand, someone else is to assess the situation the likelihood of error is even greater. The value of the life of Bartimaeus, a blind beggar in a land in which beggars were plentiful, could not be rated particularly high, yet this man was called to be healed and even some of those who discounted him may have been among those who were sent to fetch him.

The whole question of the valuation of a life is wide open to error, and inevitably the idea of expediency creeps in. Mr Norman St John Stevas is quoted as saying, 'Once a concession about the disposability of human life is made in one sphere, it will inevitably spread to others. The recognition of voluntary euthanasia by the law would, at once, be followed by pressure to extend its scope to deformed persons and imbeciles, and eventually to the old and any who could be shown to be burdens to society.'

Expediency is self-propagating. The 'thin end of the wedge' concept is not to be lightly discounted.

Practical problems
In addition to the ethical difficulties, considerable though these are, the practical difficulties must also be considered.

Who is to administer death?
The inherent relationship between the doctor and his patient is related to the accepted concept of healing and promoting recovery and health. Killing has no part in that relationship as we conceive it, and a radical change of concept would be necessary for 'killing doctors' to become an accepted idea. If such a change took place, would society demand of the doctor involved in neonatal, geriatric, or cancer-related specialities that he should be prepared to 'do' euthanasias, in the same way as the gynaecologist is currently under pressure to 'do' the other form of life termination, abortion?

If the doctor is to be involved, will this, in due course, require a specialty register of thanatologists – specialists in death?

If it is granted that the practice might be received with grave misgivings by the doctors, who else might be employed? Our veterinary colleagues, although experienced, would hardly welcome an extension of a responsibility which many of them find difficult enough when applied to animals. One cannot envisage a long queue of applicants for a special appointment in this field!

In fact, if such proposals as the euthanasia bills were to be enacted, the involvement of doctors or nurses would be inevitable, since only they would be qualified to handle such an issue, taking into account the peculiarly clinical content of such a decision.

Social implications

The social implications of voluntary euthanasia need little imagination if we consider the situations in which a patient must make a decision.

The elderly person who is beginning to feel alone, unsupported and possibly depressed, or who is beginning to feel that she is a burden to the relatives with whom she lives, would be immediately under social pressure to lift such a burden. Would this make it right?

The relatives too, might feel that it was time the old lady made up her mind and, without actually putting the idea into words might apply the same kind of subtle, or not so subtle, pressures as one already encounters in relation to application for residential or other care.

Since the event itself is irrevocable, the potential for guilt and self-recrimination for a relative who has been, even secretly, 'consenting unto' the deliberate death of a loved one is very great. One might even envisage the exchange in the midst of a 'domestic difference' between husband and wife: 'Yes, you managed to get your mother to have herself done in, but you'll have more of a job with me!' Even caring, attentive relatives who have given themselves sacrificially can feel guilty about relinquishing that care to a hospital unit, especially if the person subsequently dies from the progressing condition. What would be the load of guilt if that demise were deliberate?

Financial pressure, too, is easy to envisage. If you are in nursing home care, and are not too sure if you can afford next month's fees, might not this suggest the temptation to ask for an earlier 'exit'? Would this be acceptable in what we like to think of as a compassionate society?

Who is to decide the real motives in such a request? Who, save God himself, can look upon the heart and know what has gone on there?

Wider implications for society as a whole are also easily seen. Intolerance for the old by the younger would move easily towards the identification of a group who would be seen as having lived 'too long'. Ought they not to be lifting the economic burden which their continuing dependency is placing upon the community? The wedge is driven a little deeper as the decision has to be made for some - 'in their own interests', of course, and the move towards involuntary termination makes one more step. There is already an expressed opinion that the growing problem of dementing illness among older people will inevitably lead to the introduction of some form of non-voluntary termination of life.

The acceptance of voluntary euthanasia would be a first step in this direction. Is this a road down which we would wish to see society travel? A road which leads to the discounting of human life to such an extent that it may be considered dispensable when it no longer comes up to standard. One must ask - whose standards?

Some Christian principles
There is no Scriptural justification for the idea of mercy-killing or euthanasia. Life is clearly defined as God-given, and the length of days is equally clearly recognised as being in the hands of him who gave life itself.

The taking of life, and, in particular, the taking of innocent life, is specifically forbidden and, indeed, the only circumstances in which the taking of life is permitted are those in which judicial punishment for specific offence is involved. The personal responsibility for such an action was even avoided in Israel by the means of execution used - terrible as we may consider such a method. Stoning of an offender by a group of others made it impossible to identify the one who had thrown the fatal missile, thus laying the responsibility upon the community as a whole.

It is, however, quite interesting to observe that the call for the legalisation of the killing of the innocent ill and disabled seems to come from the same pressure groups as the plea to spare the life of the unmistakably guilty, which issued in the abolition of capital punishment.

In the Old Testament, Elijah, in the midst of his depression, not to mention his physical and emotional exhaustion, asks the Lord for 'euthanasia' - 'It is enough - take away my life!' (1 Kings 19:3). His request was not denied - it was simply ignored! He was fed, rested, ministered to, and then sent off to a further realm of fruitful service.

In the first chapter of II Samuel, an Amalekite makes the claim that he administered euthanasia to Saul in his mortally wounded state, Saul having already asked his armour-bearer to do the same for him. The response to this claim makes it quite clear that this was not an acceptable action, even in the heat of battle and in the case of severe, possibly mortal, wounds.

When we turn to the New Testament we find the Lord Jesus Christ bringing some to life from death, and bringing healing to many more, but we nowhere read of him bestowing the gift of death to a sufferer whose condition was intractable or irremediable. For him personally, death was an enemy to be finally defeated. Although it was to be the means to the glorious end - his resurrection, he did not embrace it without that horror and abhorrence which we glimpse in the Garden of Gethsemane.

We cannot dismiss that agony and the deep desire that the cup of death and the wrath of God should pass from him, as any mere formality of theology. He did not want to die - he was willing to go through with it for us and for the joy that was set before him, but this was no desired, easy way out.

While there was, and is, salvation in the death and rising again of the Lord Jesus, death offers no salvation in itself, even to those whose life is barely tolerable. Christian compassion will bring the gift of relief by all necessary means, but the 'gift of death' is not one of them.

It has been argued that, in the light of the Gospel and of the hope of eternal life after death, the Christian might embrace death as a desirable thing. The Apostle Paul seems perhaps to be suggesting such an idea when he speaks of departing to be 'with Christ, which is far better', but even he makes it plain, despite his considerable 'thorn in the flesh', that he accepts the timing of such matters as being in God's hands.

It is true that the Christian need not fear death, but nowhere is he enjoined to seek it as a means of avoiding the sufferings of a world in which persecution, distress and sickness were widely prevalent. Even in the early days of the Church, if we examine the attitudes to sufferings which were taught by the early writers they are seen as a means of grace when borne in Christ's name. There was no suggestion of an escape clause by the route of honourable suicide, or of the possibility of one brother taking another's life to spare him the forthcoming tribulation and suffering.

The sanctity of life is a principle so inherent in the whole of God's dealings with men, that it is stated only in the most general terms. 'Do not put an innocent or honest person to death, for I will not acquit the guilty.' (Ex. 23:7).

In dealing with suffering, Scripture is quite specific. It is the responsibility of the follower of Christ to be compassionate, as he is compassionate. To visit the bereaved, the imprisoned, the lonely; to give to the poor and needy and to minister to the sick. The cup of cold water given in the Lord's name is recognised as given unto him. But yet again we find no suggestion that the termination of life might be a means of compassion, in spite of the undeniable fact that the teaching of the New Testament was delivered in an age in which the means of relief of much more prevalent suffering was infinitely less than we may currently employ.

The emphasis of Scripture is on life, on the gift of life and on the eternal nature and abundance of that life. Death for the believer is not an inevitable end, but rather is the entrance into a fuller dimension of life. That entrance, however, is not determined by our deciding that the time for it has come. We are required in this matter as in all others, to place our faith and dependence upon him who faced death on our behalf. His was no euthanasia - no easy death, but its agony was purposeful and was not only an entrance, rather than an exit for him, but furnished an entrance for all who believe on him into the resurrection life which he accomplished for us.

The Christian view of death itself, as well as that of life, is a positive one, and does not include the concept of mere escape. If we accept that the grace by which we enter into such life is available to all while we live, we cannot envisage death without that grace as any kind of advantage, especially since such an exit is into a lost eternity. Can we, then, as Christians, envisage the deliberate removal of any person for whom Christ died, from what our forefathers would have called the room of grace? While life remains, the possibility of that grace also remains.

There is much, then, in terms of ethical, moral, practical, social and indeed spiritual difficulty in the concept of euthanasia or mercy-killing. In none of these areas is it, in the ultimate analysis, an easy way out, for the subject, for the doctor, for the family or for society; and, as was remarked in a seminar on this subject some years ago, 'it is to be hoped that such proposals will be allowed to die a natural death'. It does, however, seem likely that they will be resurrected in due course and, if we truly value the standards of our faith and of society, it will be necessary yet again to resist.

If we are to resist the pressures for euthanasia, it is not enough simply to be vociferous in the political, legal and ethical debate. We shall carry little credibility unless our practice matches our precept. If we believe that there is a better way to show compassion for the terminally ill and the irremedially disabled, then we must demonstrate this by high standards of professional care and by widespread personal commitment to the provision of resources for such care. It is not enough to deplore the idea of euthanasia; we must improve the care of the dying, the disabled and the disadvantaged so that the concept is redundant. Then only can society be considered compassionate and mercy will not seem to need to kill.

THE PROSPECTS FOR ETHICAL MEDICINE

Ian L. Brown

A reading of the essays in this volume must impress upon us the dramatic impact of one crucial event in the recent history of the United Kingdom – the 1967 Abortion Act. This single enactment has had an influence on our spiritual, family and societal life far beyond its legally defined terms. Various contributors refer to it and its implications, and it would not be overstating the case to say that all the issues discussed in this volume have developed rapidly as a result of this Act.

This Act was almost universally condemned by the medical profession. A letter to *The Lancet* signed by all the Presidents of the medical Royal Colleges declared it to be unnecessary. Yet it had become so indelibly written into the fabric of our society that a short time later the same group (although different individuals) could defend it in a similar letter against any modification. Here is one of the great U-turns of recent history.

This *volte face* of the leaders of the medical profession as a whole paints a dramatic picture of the 'final unravelling' of our Christian value-system in this country. Indeed, the reversal has gone so far that even Christian medical practitioners now find difficulty in maintaining a 'conservative' position on medical ethics.

This concluding chapter is an attempt to draw together the different strands of the essays collected in this volume, and to present some guidelines for the Christian assessment of medical ethics.

Dr Cameron has described cogently the decline of Christian values and conduct which flows from changes in conviction. A recent publication, *The Influence of Christians in Medicine*, begins thus:

The theme of this book is that Western Medicine, from the fourth century AD to the present day, has owed a great debt to Christianity and to individual Christians for the maintenance of its tradition and progress.[1]

This Christian Medical Fellowship publication charts the progress of medical history, describing the role of committed Christians in almost every aspect of the development and progress of medical science. From the founding of early hospitals to the development of modern scientific medicine Christians have been in the forefront. Often they have pioneered dramatic advances in social concern and improvements in the availability of medical services.

Yet we must guard against over-emphasis of this role. The secularist can also write his medical history to show the great advances which have come from the work of humanists, and it would be ludicrous to suggest that only Christians have given anything of value to the human race in medicine or any other field.

Nonetheless, Christian ethical and moral values have significantly constrained the behaviour of our society for a millenium. These values, along with its inherited Greek Hippocratic Oath have been accepted by the medical profession as the basis for its conduct. Accordingly medicine has long been regarded as a profession in which the practitioner has a 'calling', *i.e.* he or she has been drawn into it, not for personal gain, but for service to humanity.

The medical profession has therefore an inherited bias towards Christian values. This bias derives from the essentially Christian mores of our society handed down over the generations and revitalised at the Reformation and during the revivals of the eighteenth and nineteenth centuries. Many great missionary endeavours of the nineteenth century were led by doctors stirred up by the desire to heal people physically and spiritually.

However, like most inherited characteristics the resemblance to the forefather diminishes with time. As society in

1. *The Influence of Christians in Medicine*, J. T. Aitken, H. W. C. Fuller & D. Johnson (eds), London, 1984.

general has drifted from its Christian consensus so the medical profession has wavered and slipped until it now reflects a secular, post-Christian pluralist society in its attitudes. This has happened with frightening rapidity.

When the writer was a student in 1974, in a group of six doing gynaecology, all objected to assisting in a proposed abortion, unsure that the grounds were valid under the legislation. Five had no clearly definable religious convictions but all were affected by an inherited sense of ethics based on the concept that human life is of infinite value. Not one doubted that the fetus was a human person. A Christian medical student, taking that position today, might risk losing his 'class ticket' in gynaecology, without which qualification as a doctor is impossible. Experience of teaching and discussing such matters suggests that virtually none of today's students ever pauses to question the reasons given for any particular abortion. It is assumed to be legal. It is assumed to be right.

This dramatic shift in the position of the medical profession in the last 20 years is described by Dr Cameron as a change from being 'healers' to 'relievers of suffering'. While not denying that the relief of suffering is part of the healing process, and part of the healer's responsibility, it is immensely significant that this 'relief of suffering' now refers not solely to the healing of the patient (to whom the doctor is bound by his ethical code) but refers also to the relief of suffering in the relatives or even potential suffering of future generations or society at large.

In his book *The Great Evangelical Disaster* the late Francis Schaeffer wrote thus:

> We live in a society today where all things are relative and the final value is whatever makes the individual or society 'happy' or feel good at the moment . . . . This is even true with regard to human life.[2]

2. *The Great Evangelical Disaster*, F. A. Schaeffer, Eastbourne, 1985.

Semantic expansion has also given us a new concept of 'compassion', an emotional response which depends on the dignity of the sufferer for its very existence. Compassion also may be extrapolated from the individual patient to his family and to society as a whole. This may then result in the killing of a fetus in order to exhibit compassion for the mother, family or wider society.

Against this background James Philip presents the Biblical perspective on the sanctity of the individual human life, seeing in the doctrine of creation, the Mosaic legislation and the New Testament the infinite value of mankind 'bought with a price'.

This principle is the very essence of all the contributions to this volume. For this we make no apology, our purpose being to assess moral and ethical dilemmas in current medical practice in the light of the basic teaching of Scripture.

It is the conviction of the contributors to this volume that we as a society have lost all sense of the special nature of the human person, precisely because we have wandered from the basic assumption that all life is a gift from God, a gift whose value is indelibly underlined by the adding of redemption to creation: 'You are not your own, for you are bought with a price.'

Unfortunately it is not just society at large that has lost this sense, but the Church and individual Christians have been affected too. Our society once drew its strength, its 'moral fibre', from the basic tenets of Christianity. We now live in a pluralist society where men of all faiths and no faith co-exist. After a century of liberal teaching the Church no longer speaks with convincing authority on moral issues *i.e.* authority which stems not from ecclesiastical structures but from the Word of God. The individual Christian is uncertain about these issues because the Church is uncertain (*e.g.* within the Church of Scotland, a General Assembly decision on abortion was reversed at the following Assembly). Moreover the individual is unhappy because he is uncertain about the 'fairness' of establishing absolutes from a Scripture which he is told by theologians is flawed, contradictory and written in a different social milieu from his own.

IVF . . . antenatal diagnosis . . . embryo research. What can Scripture say? Its writers knew nothing of these techniques. Yet Scripture does deal with these issues. It is God-breathed and as such is all sufficient for our purposes. We need confidence in its truthfulness and boldness in its application.

The remaining essays deal with the practical issues of genetic engineering, IVF, embryo research, abortion, the care of the handicapped newborn and euthanasia. Much has been written about these issues elsewhere, by Christian and non-Christian alike. The crucial issue is surely the concept of the 'non-person'. Francis Schaeffer and Everett Koop were the first to emphasise, in *Whatever Happened to the Human Race?*,[3] the slippery slope of change in social conditions in pre-1939 Germany which allowed for the elimination of socially unacceptable groups, namely gypsies, mixed race people, the handicapped and mentally ill; in short, all who were not contributing in economic terms to society. This of course was a society preparing for world conquest, and the war effort required 100% commitment. The Holocaust of the Jewish extermination camps followed initial steps to purify the nation taken in these pre-war days. It was possible only as a result of the classification of certain groups as 'non-persons' as far as the state was concerned. Once the concept of 'non-persons' was established, the slide into human experimentation was logical if not inevitable.

No-one today would dare to categorise any group as 'non-persons'. Or would they? In effect that is what the Warnock Report does – before 14 days' gestation the embryo is not a human being, not a person. It may, therefore, be used as an experimental object. That is what the Abortion Act does by allowing us the opportunity to dispense with the intra-uterine 'product of conception' with often minimal reason.

3. *Whatever Happened to the Human Race?*, F. A. Schaeffer & C. E. Koop, London, 1980.

That is what may be done in the neonatal unit if a defective baby is born – though withholding food and water in the name of 'compassion' is a distortion of language so bizarre that even the 'alternative' comedians of today might shrink from using it. That too is what may be done in the geriatric unit when the elderly become disorientated, incontinent, and a burden on society.

What guidelines are there for Christians in the debate on medical ethics?

First, the Bible is our rule and guidebook in these as in all other matters. The Biblical principle that man is created in God's image, and has been bought at the infinite price of Christ's death on the cross must pervade all our thinking. Every aspect of life must be brought under the authority of God's word to us. Clearly we will not find a verse dealing explicitly with IVF, but in this, as in all, we must look for Biblical principles to apply, and then we must submit our human inclinations to what we find.

Secondly, we must be awake and aware of what is happening in the world around us. In 1967 the churches were asleep when the Abortion Act was passed, and only those in favour of the legislation were really clear about what was being planned.

Thirdly, we have a responsibility to God and to future generations in our stewardship of life – both our own lives, and our corporate life.

Fourthly, we must not be pressurised by the world view which holds that since we live in a pluralist society we must modify our convictions in line with those being propagated around us:

> Therefore, I urge you, brothers, in view of God's mercy, to offer your bodies as living sacrifices, holy and pleasing to God – which is your spiritual worship. Do not conform any longer to the pattern of this world, but be transformed by the renewing of your mind. Then you will be able to test and approve what God's will is – his good, pleasing and perfect will.
>
> Romans 12:1,2

Ian Brown

What are the prospects for medicine that stands within the great Western ethical tradition of Hippocrates and the Christian faith? There can be no doubt that they seem bleak, since medicine has largely chosen to follow the path of the secular values of our society. But there has never been a clearer role for Christian medicine to play, standing in prophetic witness to the great tradition, and seeking to call the profession back to its roots. Let us pray that we may not shirk this responsibility, but will have the perception and the courage that we need.

126

INDEX